gentle dying

The simple guide to achieving a peaceful death

Felicity Warner

HAY HOUSE

Australia • Canada • Hong Kong • India
South Africa • United Kingdom • United States

First published and distributed in the United Kingdom by:
Hay House UK Ltd, 292B Kensal Rd, London W10 5BE. Tel.: (44) 20 8962 1230;
Fax: (44) 20 8962 1239. www.hayhouse.co.uk

Published and distributed in the United States of America by:
Hay House, Inc., PO Box 5100, Carlsbad, CA 92018-5100. Tel.: (1) 760 431 7695 or
(800) 654 5126; Fax: (1) 760 431 6948 or (800) 650 5115. www.hayhouse.com

Published and distributed in Australia by:
Hay House Australia Ltd, 18/36 Ralph St, Alexandria NSW 2015.
Tel.: (61) 2 9669 4299; Fax: (61) 2 9669 4144. www.hayhouse.com.au

Published and distributed in the Republic of South Africa by:
Hay House SA (Pty), Ltd, PO Box 990, Witkoppen 2068. Tel./Fax: (27) 11 467 8904.
www.hayhouse.co.za

Published and distributed in India by:
Hay House Publishers India, Muskaan Complex, Plot No.3, B-2, Vasant Kunj,
New Delhi – 110 070. Tel.: (91) 11 4176 1620; Fax: (91) 11 4176 1630.
www.hayhouse.co.in

Distributed in Canada by:
Raincoast, 9050 Shaughnessy St, Vancouver, BC V6P 6E5. Tel.: (1) 604 323 7100;
Fax: (1) 604 323 2600

A catalogue record for this book is available from the British Library.

ISBN 978-1-84850-005-1

Printed and bound in Great Britain by TJ International, Padstow

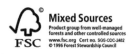

Mixed Sources
Product group from well-managed
forests and other controlled sources
www.fsc.org Cert no. SGS-COC-2482
© 1996 Forest Stewardship Council

gentle dying

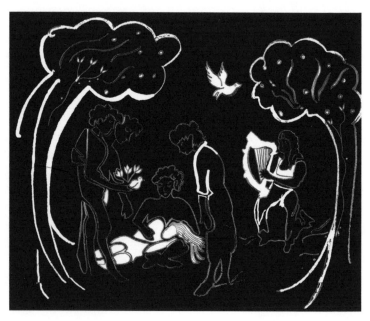

A Gentle Death by Lusea Warner

To Thelma

And those, too numerous to mention, who invited me
with such trust to journey with them

*The journey between life and death flows peacefully
as a slowly winding river.*

Basho

CONTENTS

PREFACE

If you've ever sat helplessly with someone who is dying and wished that you could do something positive to help them, then this book is for you.

When our final days come, most of us aren't sure what to expect. Throughout our lives most of us postpone getting to grips with this issue. But if at this stage, while we are fit, we can acquire our best understanding of just what happens as the death process unfolds, this will lessen our worries. And if we've explored the options well ahead of time, we will feel more empowered, as we die, to request and receive the best care possible for our body, mind and spirit.

You may be flicking through these pages to find out what a gentle death is, or perhaps you are a partner, lover, brother or sister or friend of someone who has just learned that his or her life will soon be ending.

This guide will tell you how to help someone to die peacefully once medicine has reached its limits and when human touch can become a greater help than hard-edged medicine. You'll find practical information on using therapeutic touch, therapeutic sound, and simple breathing techniques as well as meditation and a host of other simple but safe methods to help not only those close to death but also those who are caring for them.

This guide also explores spiritual and psychological issues and advises on how to be a good companion to someone who is dying. Understanding what happens in the last stages of life is in many ways a vital part of helping someone towards a peaceful death. Pregnant women are encouraged to make birth plans stating their wishes before going into labour. You can do the same at the end of life, ensuring that it's as good an experience as you'd wish it to be.

Giving love and time to someone who is nearing the end of their life will bring untold miracles including:

- helping them to die with peace and dignity

- helping them to dissolve fears and feel safe

- ensuring that dying is a sacred rite of passage and that their life has been worthwhile

- ensuring that they have felt loved and supported right up until their very last breath.

The love and care that we can give at the end of life are among the most precious gifts that we can ever share with one another.

INTRODUCTION

People are shocked when they hear that I help people to ... die.

'What do you mean ... you help people die? What you do exactly?' they ask, looking anxious.

'Isn't dying best left to the doctors who do a great job, despite difficult conditions? After all, they've got drugs and technology.'

'Aren't people best left alone to die, as long as they aren't suffering?'

'Why would anyone want to do such a weird thing with their life? Being with dying people must be really horrible and upsetting, no? Doesn't it make you depressed?'

It's true, I am not a doctor or a nurse. Neither am I a trained care worker. I don't seek to duplicate these professionals' work. I work alongside them. I have great respect for all they do, and they — increasingly frequently — respect what I do.

My approach is completely different from theirs. My skills have nothing to do with machines or chemicals — in fact, just the opposite. The tools of my trade are all much more human — namely my voice, my hands and, more importantly, an open and loving heart.

I can help people to die well in any setting, whether it be in hospitals, care homes, hospices or in the dying person's own home — and I begin my role when the doctors have done all that they can.

My work fits in alongside whatever treatment is in progress. I aim to make the atmosphere around the dying person serene and safe to enable him or her to let go quietly, when he or she feels ready. It's an ancient and very human way of helping people die rather than any strictly medical one.

People don't realize that dying can take a long time and that it can be such a very lonely process.

All the best treatment and medicine in the world aren't going to keep someone alive when their time has truly come. Therefore switching the focus from trying to make them better to making them feel comfortable and safe is a wonderful way of honouring the end of life.

Controlling pain and all the other distressing symptoms is of course very important, but the heavy-handed use of drugs may mask the dying experience, robbing the person of the full richness and revelations that can occur. A gentle death, which is what we all hope for, can be achieved by combining the best care that medicine can provide alongside other subtler methods such as massage, visualization, breathing techniques and other holistic ways of calming and soothing. By using these, the amount of drugs required may be reduced, helping the person to feel more in touch with what's happening and also more in control of their own wellbeing.

Death is very similar to birth. It isn't, as some think, just the moment immediately before your heart stops beating or when you take your last breath. It's usually a slow and gentle unravelling process. It involves a process akin to birth labour. There is a series of important and diverse stages which affect emotional and spiritual levels over and above the purely physical process most people are more familiar with.

There is no ideal place to die, although home is often most desirable. Hospitals are busy and noisy and are focused on curing disease. Hospices and care homes, however good, can be institutional and impersonal. The dying need a tranquil atmosphere with soft lighting and soothing sounds in order to feel supported on their journey.

Working with the dying can, of course, be very sad. It can also be very moving at times. Often it can be surprisingly funny and joyful. Some say that it can be the source of the richest blessings imaginable. It is certainly the greatest privilege to help someone die well and make them feel that somehow their life is complete and has been worthwhile and that they have been truly loved.

After hundreds of thousands of years of human evolution, why does the thought of dying still frighten us so much, and why is this fear actually increasing as time passes?

These questions puzzled me when I worked as a health journalist and was engaged in writing a series of articles about people facing death through terminal illness. Many of them were young, with small children, and were having to learn to live with the fact that life had somehow, and through no fault of their own, sold them short. They were all, coincidentally, women, and the majority of them had cancer.

They hoped that by telling their stories, their experiences would be able to help others who might find themselves in the same harrowing situation.

Most of them were very ill, but were still determined to live for the moment and make the most of what time they had left. The interviews often lasted for several hours — there'd be breaks while we waited for their painkillers to work and, while we waited, we chatted. I remember one asking me if I could help her rearrange the shunt that she had in her chest which was draining fluid from her lung. It had got tangled up in her bra strap.

Another one asked me if I would like to feel the tumour in her groin, as she couldn't find a way of describing it. I'd never seen a tumour before, and while I hesitantly ran my finger over it, her four-year-old daughter offered me some Smarties and asked cheerfully if I had cancer too. If so, where was it?

These women were amazingly cheerful but they were all, hardly surprisingly, very frightened and anxious about what was eventually going to happen to them. In between treatments they were determined to carry on as usual with the daily routines of caring for their children, getting the shopping and also making plans ahead of time for when they knew that they wouldn't be there any more. Their main fears weren't for themselves, but for those that they were going to leave behind — partners, young children, elderly parents, close friends and all the people they knew and loved. Several of them even cooked meals to leave in the freezer, knowing that the food would come in handy once they had died.

We spent many hours in conversation, compiling the information to put the feature together. I got used to discussing diagnosis and treatment plans and also to asking them about their remaining hopes, fears and dreams. The most interesting part of their story always came once I'd put my notebook away and we were sharing a post-interview cup of tea.

Relaxing and letting go at last, they'd all say how good it was to — as one of them put it — 'talk dirty' about dying to a complete stranger, who listened and wasn't upset or squeamish, and didn't try to give them advice.

Although it was tough, for them and me, they were relieved to be able to use words like 'death' and 'dying' and not feel guilty about it.

I was astonished as they told me about their lives and how it felt to know that they were dying, and to learn just how lonely and isolated they felt.

Their friends and relatives were becoming increasingly distant from them and were refusing to engage with or acknowledge the reality of the situation. Although these friends would still telephone, their talk was usually full of false optimism. There'd be many conversations along the lines of 'Soon you'll be getting better' and 'Why don't we plan a treat for when you've got over all this?' A good proportion of my interviewees, sadly, were rapidly becoming disconnected from everyone they felt close to.

A good example was Sarah, an accountant in her thirties, who told me that her own mother was so furious with her for getting an untreatable form of breast cancer that she wasn't speaking to her any more.

Diana, an actress also in her thirties, told me that the despair from not being able to share her thoughts with anyone always hit her in the middle of the night when the family was asleep. She'd creep downstairs to the kitchen, pour a glass of wine and sob, with the dog on her lap for company.

They were all comforted by the fact that I clearly wasn't scared of talking to them about dying. This was because in my own life I had lost two very close family members. This had happened when I was in my teens and at a particularly vulnerable stage in my life.

The first was my grandmother, with whom I had lived since the age of six after my parents divorced. The second was my stepfather, who died suddenly, and at a very young age, from a fatal heart attack. The shock and turbulence stemming from both these events led me, after much soul-searching, towards a very focused spiritual and healing path that helped me to create a personal philosophy about life and death, as well as to develop a set of skills in dealing with trauma. These skills, for me, are still evolving.

As their illnesses progressed, nearly all of these women spoke of a need to prepare themselves emotionally and spiritually for what lay ahead, in order to bring some meaning to what was happening to them. They also wanted to make their deaths somehow inspirational, to soften the loss and bring a positive glow to the memories of those they were leaving behind. Between them they left a wonderful collection of poems, drawings, booklets for their children, pottery and even videos.

Most of them were strengthened by receiving complementary therapies, and loved having aromatherapy massage or reflexology treatments. These made them feel touchable and human again. During my visits, as we became closer, I'd massage them with essential oils, or bring my Tibetan 'singing bowls' for them to play and enjoy.

The greatest privilege of all came when three of them asked me to be at their death and to help ease them along by singing and giving them healing, even when they were unconscious.

Working with these pioneering women was an extraordinary time. It now seems no coincidence that many of them were very creative — writers, musicians, artists and actors. They all had the vision, although none of them actually met each other, to want their deaths to be beautiful, dignified and inspiring to others.

This has encouraged me to develop what they unknowingly began — a desire to re-vision the way that we deal with death and dying, and the need for compassionate and holistic care in the final stages of life.

I became a volunteer at a local hospice, enrolled on a counselling course and honed my own healing and intuitive skills. I also did some research to find out how other cultures, now and throughout history, have helped members of their community to die. I realized that a huge body of knowledge about helping people to die had been lost — it had always belonged to the community and needed to be returned again.

I also trawled every faith and religion, spoke to people who deal with death every day and talked to many experts — doctors, priests, nurses, mediums, shamen, nuns and complementary therapists. I discovered that, although they all had their own approaches, there wasn't any integration of ideas or practices towards creating a modern paradigm. It seemed that no one was thinking outside the box.

Gradually my ideas began to grow and eventually led me into setting up a project called The Hospice of the Heart, the world's first Internet-based hospice dedicated to providing help, advice, information and inspiration on death and dying. I also started to give seminars, workshops and classes on dying well and creating support networks.

The Hospice of the Heart is now a registered UK charity with a vibrant global community of people dedicated to making death a better experience. We also teach carers, and the wider public, a method called Gentle Dying which uses all the holistic skills described in this book. It can be learned in a day and used by anyone — it is so simple and can help anyone to achieve a peaceful and gentle death, wherever they are.

I also teach an increasing number of people who wish to work as 'soul midwives' and midwives to the dying. They support people on a soul level as they cross the sacred threshold between this life and the next. They are a growing band of exceptional people and are taking this work out into their community and making a significant difference to the lives — and deaths — of everyone they help.

CHAPTER ONE
A Gentle Unravelling

Death is usually a process rather than an event. It's the gradual unravelling of a life, and a slow and gentle letting-go, like a feather taking off in the wind.

Sometimes death is the result of an accident or sudden illness. Even then, the final and fleeting moments may have a surprising grace of their own.

Apart from the obvious physical aspects endured as the body winds down, death is a process that profoundly affects our inner being, emotions and psyche on many levels. Dying is a time that many of us think of as being the end, but it's also often a beginning, when the inner life can unexpectedly begin to blossom.

Dying is an intimate and sacred journey best done in its own time, in a tranquil and peaceful way. When it goes well, it's an honouring of a life well lived and an important rite of passage.

The experience of dying, although similar in all of us, follows a highly individual route. We tend to die as we have lived — some with cheerful optimism, others with fear or boiling rage. We all die in our own unique way.

If our passing is gentle and meaningful, it can be a graceful and exalted experience for us and our families, and those left behind sometimes look back and see it as an event that healed family rifts, enabling people to reconnect with each other in a way that is positively life-changing for everyone involved.

Indeed, anyone who has witnessed a good death will tell you of the wonderful sense of awe it evokes, which is similar in so many ways to the emotions we experience and sense of wonderment that we feel when a baby is born.

Birth and death, the two great opposites, share startling similarities.

Not so long ago when people were born and died in their own homes, arriving and departing were community events with friends gathering and supporting the families. Towns and villages had midwives and 'wise women' who were skilled in the art of birth and death, providing practical help and comfort.

In those days, everyone was used to seeing, hearing, smelling and knowing about death as well as preparing for new life.

When people used to die in their own beds with their families around them, enveloped in the safe hub of family life, the family were at ease, aware of the natural course of illness and death and supported by their friends and neighbours.

The fear of dying has increased as people die away from home and in hospital or in other unfamiliar surroundings. Smoothing away the fear and replacing it with loving care is one of the first important steps towards a gentle death.

More of us are now choosing to die at home, but this can only happen if we have family and friends who are able to support us. Good pain relief is one of the greatest attributes of modern medicine, but we mustn't forget to add affection and time and love. Miracles happen when people feel safe and nurtured. In helping people to die well, a kind heart is as valuable as medical training, because it is the source of happiness for both oneself and others.

It is a parting gift we can give our loved ones, and by improving the deaths of everyone around us we will ultimately improve our own.

Gentle Dying

'We're sorry, but there is nothing more that can be done.' This is what we are often told. It's one of the bluntest pieces of news we may ever have to receive. It leaves us without any sense of hope at all.

Knowing that someone you love is going to die is bad enough, but feeling that there is nothing you can do to make their passing a good one puts us in a very bleak dilemma — and it's a dilemma faced by thousands of us around the world every day.

Gentle dying is all about helping people to die in the best possible way for them. It may simply involve holding their hand and just being there with a warm and open heart. Or it may involve quietly reading them one of their favourite poems, massaging their arm, stroking their forehead or lying beside them and swaddling them with soft blankets.

If you find yourself sitting beside someone whose life is slipping away, I hope you'll be inspired to try out some of these simple techniques and help them both embrace and experience death in a compassionate, gentle and ultimately healing way.

When we arrive in this world we are greeted, loved and welcomed by our parents, siblings, grandparents and friends. Everyone celebrates and opens their hearts to us. We are cuddled, cherished and adored. Our very presence celebrates the miracle of life.

But when we die, the story is often so different.

Most of us die away from home — in a hospital, rest home or hospice, cared for by kindly but busy strangers. Sadly, many of us die alone in unfamiliar surroundings that bring no atmosphere of love or comfort.

Helping people to die gently, with a sense of grace and dignity, is much easier than it sounds. By using any of the suggestions in this book you can make a difference, whatever your surroundings.

In ancient times the act of dying was regarded as a time of spiritual preparation for whatever lay ahead. The priests and healers tending the dying were initiates into the great mysteries of life and were skilled experts in treating the body, mind and soul. Their understanding and knowledge were so refined that each part of the dying process was perfectly understood and managed, ensuring that death came peacefully and with a recognition of its sacred meaning.

The sick were tended in tranquil temples, so different from our modern hospitals, where the sound of water soothed their emotions, and scented herbs and oils anointed their bodies.

This knowledge is gradually and once again being remembered and brought back into use.

What Is a Gentle Death?

Last year I visited my friend John who was in a coma following a heart attack. He was being cared for in an intensive-care unit and was wired up to an army of whirring machines which watched every minute sign of life in his body.

The flashing monitors were connected by electrodes to his chest and scalp. They showed that his heartbeat, brain activity, oxygen content in his lungs and levels of vital hormones were all hanging by a thread. Even if he did wake up from this terrible trauma and survive, he would never be able to see, hear, talk or move by himself again.

We all knew this, and the doctors confirmed it, and yet a good and peaceful death was never considered to be an option — the fight for life in this hi-tech unit was the driving force behind John's care. To lose the battle would be seen as a failure by the medics. As John slowly slipped away, looking like a piece of meat on a butcher's block, no one was encouraged to comfort him, hold his hand or stroke his cheek, let alone whisper any soothing words of kindness or love in his ear. He died surrounded by experts and millions of pounds' worth of equipment, but untouched by human hands.

John's death sounds extreme, but it's common enough. Cold and lacking in any tenderness.

Yet my friend Marianne's death was a totally different experience.

I visited her on the day before she died. She was upstairs in her own bed, covered in a soft quilt that she had made herself many years ago from the outgrown frocks of her daughters. The quilt, to Marianne, contained so many loving memories.

John Taverner's exquisite and ethereal music — The Protecting Veil — played in her bedroom, which was softly lit by candles. Her sister Serena had flown over from Australia and was massaging her feet with rose oil, the smell of which filled the room — which seemed for at least a moment to have the air of an exotic Moorish palace.

Another friend, Charlie, arrived to give Marianne a further sound experience in the form of what he called a 'sound bath'. He played Celtic airs on a small harp. Her pain was eased. Her troubled breathing became more relaxed. Downstairs, delicious food was being prepared amidst much laughter and more music.

Many whom Marianne loved were there keeping vigil around her bed through what turned out to be her very peaceful last hours. It was a gentle and loving death, and although she was mourned, her friends celebrated her life to the full as she died.

They watched over her and enriched her to the end.

The Perfect Way to Go

Today is a good day to die,
for all the things of my life are present.
Native American saying

Most of us have a slightly romantic picture in our minds of how we would like death to be. It would probably be at home, in our own bed (with the cat at the foot of it), pain-free and surrounded by our loved ones.

This is probably one of the most perfect ways to go, but unless we spend just a little time thinking about it, while we are still well, the chances of it turning out like this are slim.

Statistics show that although 70 per cent of us would like to die at home, in reality only around 17 per cent of us actually achieve this. The majority of us end our days in hospital, a care home or a hospice, where we place our care and wellbeing in the hands of strangers.

Obviously, sudden deaths are impossible to plan for, but given time and preparation we can put in place ideas and instructions so that everything is just how we'd like it to be.

Exploring the following ideas might help you begin to get ideas about planning for a good death — or, at least, to get you and your loved ones talking about what's important to you and also what's important for them.

How would you prioritize the following considerations on a scale of one to ten?

- to know when death is coming and what to expect

- to have someone with you (unless you prefer to die alone)

- *to be able to make decisions regarding treatment*

- *to have dignity, confidentiality and privacy*

- *to have access to hospice-quality pain relief and other symptom control, wherever you die*

- *to be able to choose where death will happen (hospital or home), to refuse treatment if you want to, and, if you choose after any treatment, to be brought home again to die*

- *to have access to up-to-date information and expertise*

- *to be spiritually and emotionally supported*

- *to choose who will be present*

- *to be able to issue advance directives such as rejecting certain treatments including blood transfusions, heart stimulants, etc. in accordance with your wishes*

- *to have time to say goodbye*

- *to be able to leave when it is time to go, and not to have life prolonged pointlessly*

- *to retain the right to fast as death approaches, and not be artificially fed or hydrated.*

Write your ideas down, then give a copy to your next of kin, doctor and lawyer. Carry a card in your wallet or purse which notifies people that you have written down what you want and where to find it.

When you were born, you cried and the world rejoiced. Live your life in a manner so that when you die the world cries and you rejoice.

Native American proverb

Imagining Your Own Death

Practical considerations play a big part in planning

for a good death. But now it's time to imagine creatively how we'd really like it to be if we could only choose.

This will show you what can be possible. The answer is 'Quite a lot!'

I had a conversation, many years ago, with a woman called Pat who was a wonderful healer and medium. She was in her late eighties. She told me glowingly and with a mischievous chuckle that she had absolutely no fear of dying, as she had already chosen what would happen and had been 'allowed' to have a sneak preview in her dreams.

She explained,

My guides were old friends to me, having worked with me all my life. During meditation one day I was invited, by Kwan Yin, the Goddess of Compassion, to choose what sort of death I'd like. I really wasn't sure and so I was invited to review all the options and scenarios and see the outcome of each one. It didn't take me long to work out that I'd like to die peacefully in my sleep outside in the garden. That night, as I slept, I was shown exactly how it would be — and when I woke up I felt utterly at peace and filled with a sense of bliss.

Just a couple of years later I had a telephone call from the retirement home where Pat had later moved to say that she had died very peacefully in her sleep in a chair, after afternoon tea in the rose garden.

She'd also left a note in her diary, found a couple of weeks later, saying 'Death isn't the end — it's just a change of address.'

I'm always astonished at how imaginative people become in my 'How to Have a Good Death' workshops. The workshops are attended by people of all backgrounds and of all ages. They are always light-hearted and jolly. Against this background they come up with some very serious plans and solutions.

After exploring what death actually means to them personally, the participants split up into groups of four or five and imagine the time, place and props they might need. There's always much laughter as the suggestions are read out. Going off in a hot-air balloon, sailing out to sea in a punt, going off in a giant firework display. These are some of the favourites. One vivacious lady in her late seventies shocked everyone by saying she wanted to die in the arms of her lover (20 years her junior), drinking champagne!

BUDDHIST PRACTICE

When Buddhist monks begin their long and arduous training, they are required to spend many months meditating on their own deaths as a way of understanding the nature of immortality and reincarnation.

As part of this practice they spend days and nights in cemeteries, alone and surrounded by the remains of the dead. While they live and sleep among the tombs, they have to visualize every detail of their dying and eventual decomposition. Eventually, they reach a point of total acceptance about the impermanence of our physical bodies and, in doing so, conquer all fear of death.

This practice is a bit extreme for most of us, but a simpler version, done comfortably at home either on our own or with a group, can enrich our understanding of how it feels to die and also how it might feel if our time is growing shorter. It can also strengthen our inner psychic tools for coping with death.

Only do this exercise when you are feeling upbeat, buoyant and centred — and don't forget: thinking about death isn't going to kill you!

Imagining Your Own Death Exercise

Set aside around 45 minutes, unplug the phone and sit or lie down comfortably.

Close your eyes and concentrate on your breathing, taking 15 slow in- and out-breaths to calm your mind.

Tell yourself, 'I am quietly and gently and peacefully slipping between two worlds. I am at peace, without pain and surrounded by love. I have no fear or anguish about the journey I am about to take.'

Then ask yourself, 'Where would I most like to die? At home in my own bed? At the home of a friend or relative? In a hospice? In a hospital or care home? Outdoors? Beside the sea? In a chair or on a sofa, on soft squishy cushions in front of a blazing log fire, on a padded reclining chair in the garden, on a blanket under a favourite tree, beside a river or stream, on an airbed on the sea, or maybe lying in a field of gently blowing wheat?

'Would I like to be on my own or would I like there to be someone with me? Would I like them to be silent, or to speak or sing to me gently? Would I like them to hold my hand or lightly stroke my hand or arm?

'What would I like to hear, smell or touch? Would I like to be wrapped up warm and swaddled with soft fabrics, or would I like to feel the lightest covering over me and a breeze across my face?'

Imagine the setting, relax your body, feel serenity ooze over you. Imagine that you are in a very favourite place, warm and comfortable and feeling peaceful and ready to let go.

When you are ready, return to normality and write down any ideas or sensations that came into your mind.

Of course, none of us can really know for sure when death will visit.

On the 'shopping list' there are quick deaths such as accidents, heart attacks, fatal strokes, asthma attacks or allergic reactions, moderately quick deaths including certain cancers, lingering deaths from chronic disease and, most commonly, the complications of old age, including pneumonia and fractures.

Imagining your own death can be a liberating experience. In other parts of the world, such as India — where death is far more integrated with daily life — it's quite normal to have some plans in place and to tell others about them.

Taking this idea one step further, lots of people like to imagine what their funerals will be like and often make elaborate plans for them well in advance — a church filled with the people we have enjoyed sharing our lives with, a moving service where our favourite music rolls out like Desert Island Discs …

moving eulogies, poems and readings by a few chosen friends, followed by a fantastic party afterwards. Or perhaps a procession to a woodland cemetery with songs and inspirational readings out in the open air followed by a ceilidh in a barn or pub. Or ... a service in a beautiful house with everyone dressed in their finest, sipping champagne cocktails before a delicious banquet (decided on and paid for by you in advance). Here again, let your imagination run riot.

Learn to die and thou shall learn how to live.
There shall none learn how to live that has not learned to die.
Tibetan Book of the Dead

What Death Teaches Us

Eric Carle's book *The Very Hungry Caterpillar* tells the story of a bright green caterpillar munching its way through huge quantities of ice cream, water melon and salami, and its gloriously greedy appetite for life. Then one day it pupates, becomes a chrysalis and lies dormant for a while before morphing into a beautiful butterfly.

As well as being a great and simple analogy for death and transfiguration, the butterfly, an age-old symbol of transformation, takes us through the mystery of shape-shifting and metamorphosis and shows us that death is just part of a continuing cycle.

As Sogyal Rinpoche explains in his *Tibetan Book of Living and Dying*, 'according to the wisdom of Buddha, we can actually use our lives to prepare for death.'

We don't have to wait for the painful death of someone close to us, or the shock of terminal illness, to force us into looking at our lives. Nor are we condemned to go out empty-handed towards death to meet the unknown. We can begin, here and now, to find meaning in our lives. We can make of every moment an opportunity to change and to prepare — wholeheartedly, precisely, and with peace of mind — for both death and eternity.

The Buddhist Bardo teachings tell us that unless we are comfortable with the idea of death, and all it implies, we won't be able to enjoy our lives fully. Embracing death and its unlimited boundless freedom should be our life's most important work. Knowing that we will all die one day focuses the need to live in the present. If we can begin to master this we can die like a newborn baby, free of all worries and fear.

Life and death are an infinite continuum where death is simply the beginning of another chapter of life, and at the same time death is a mirror in which the entire meaning of our life is reflected back to us.

Death by Choice

Sometimes death comes by our own hand and invitation. We can never know the full story or facts behind the reasons for anyone taking this decision. But I believe that we are the owners of our own destiny, so how can the choice to take our life away by our own hands be morally wrong? Or be judged harshly by others? Shouldn't we honour the decision and create a loving space around the soul that has chosen to go, for whatever reason?

Taking one's own life is often the result of a major conflict between the soul's needs and the ongoing struggle to resolve them. Not only does the soul have its own agenda, but it also has its own deep wisdom and knowingness and perfect sense of timing according to the greater divine plan.

We cannot possibly know the wider picture of someone's destiny, or the tormented inner landscape of someone in the hours before their action. Nor can we understand the karmic burdens they are carrying, the soul wounds they bear and the precise impetus that brought them to their decision ... but we do know of the grand intelligence of the soul.

Shock, anger, extreme despair, feelings of betrayal and of having let someone down are often the emotions of those left behind.

In the past, a blemish has been cast on those who've made this choice, by branding it a sin against God. But I think most soul workers would agree that God, or the wise beings, help people die from suicide in just the same unconditionally loving way that He or they help everyone else.

Some people believe that all deaths are indeed an act of suicide — a decision to go — and that we all choose the time of our dying when all is in place and all is complete.

Working with souls who have taken their lives can be a fragile and heart-rending experience. As a psychopomp (guider of souls), I am sometimes aware of a deep, dull, darkened presence nudging me, trying to talk. It feels as if it is speaking from the depths of a very deep hole, in a confined place of darkness. On a psychic level many people who commit suicide are similar to those who have died very suddenly and don't realize that they are actually dead. They can be very frightened, disorientated, frustrated and feeling trapped. It's important to tell them that you are able to help them to find their way towards the light.

If you find yourself drawn to help souls such as these, check first that you are feeling both grounded and safe. Comfort them and talk to them as if they are physically present, and explain that they will have the chance to put things right and release themselves from guilt and blame. Then lead them to the light and walk them home as you would any other person who has passed across, and ask for someone to meet them.

CHAPTER TWO
Feel Love ... and Fear Not

When Dylan Thomas urged, 'Do not go gentle into that good night ... rage, rage, against the dying of the light,' he touched on one of our greatest fears.

Instead of seeing death as a gentle surrender, he saw it as the final battle of life, a defeat of the spirit and a bitter loss of everything we hold dear. This reflects the widespread and modern view that death is, in all ways, terrifying.

The dread of losing forever those we love brings unfathomable grief, sorrow and pain.

Yet, as Richard Reoch notes in his book *Dying Well*,

> *The fear of death has an irresistible magnetism. We are drawn to it, motivated by it and appalled by it. Its power over us is fundamental to our existence. It triggers our entire nervous system at even the slightest threat and, moment after moment, it drives the life functions of our internal organs.*

For many of us the fear of death has many guises — for instance the fear of losing our 'self' — where do we go? What becomes of us? Will we feel lost and alone? And how will those we leave behind manage when we are gone? Will pain overwhelm us? Will we lose our dignity in front of others? Will we be judged for things that we now regret? Might we be punished ... in this life or the next?

The most overwhelming aspect of our fears often centres around the idea that we will sink into oblivion, a black, airless depth of nothingness.

In the West we have a deep mistrust and anxiety regarding voids and empty vacuums. We fill our lives up, packing every hour with stimulating experiences, trying at all costs to prevent nothingness and silence from creeping in. But if nothingness really worries you, think back to a time, perhaps the year before you were born, to when you weren't here. Do you miss it?

As soul companions we can sit and listen and reassure, but it is not our place to fix or rescue. Shallow reassurances and avoidance of difficult issues have no place in this work. If your friend has fears, encourage him or her to share them if they can. If the fears can't be resolved, they can at least be heard — witnessed, in a sense — and perhaps put to rest. If even this seems too difficult, light a candle and 'offer the fears up' to be solved by the force of universal good.

Creating our own good 'philosophy' about death and addressing the big thoughts from the safety of our own inner world, while we are still well, certainly gives us strength when helping others.

Some say that facing these fears is an essential part of dying, and that from working through them we may reach a stronger and safer place. Death is so much a matter of perspective — its illusionary nature can provide us with pertinent clues about the extraordinary nature of life.

Within our lives we are continually experiencing losses, some great and some small. The challenge of this is to greet each change with an attitude of acceptance and to live our lives in the present without regretting or hankering after the past or fearing the future. Death is one of these changes, simply a shift into the next phase. As the Danish philosopher Kierkegaard said, 'Life must be lived forward, but can only be understood backwards.'

We are constantly in flux.

If someone is having real difficulties in *letting go*, help them reflect on the innumerable deaths that all of us encounter over a lifetime — our babyhood, starting school, how we slowly morphed into becoming teenagers and so on — until we can look back over a lifetime of stages and almost separate identities that were definitely 'us' but faded and adjusted until we became who we are now.

Fear is nothing to be ashamed of. Even experienced professionals admit to having days when an un-anticipated situation or scenario has thrown full light onto one of their own hidden demons. The fears of the dying can unwelcomingly magnify our own and they may unexpectedly leap out of the shadows at us. It certainly helps us if we have come to peaceful terms with our own mortality when we sit with someone who is close to the end.

Working at Heart Level

It's so much easier to help someone to die gently if there is a bond of trust and empathy between you both, but it can take years to create this level of intimacy — and when someone is dying, time might be very short.

If you are a carer who is reading this, you'll know how important it is to be able to reach this deep level of trust, where each feels comfortable and completely at ease with the other.

One of the most powerful techniques that soul midwives use is creating a heart—soul connection with someone.

If you are a reflexologist or aromatherapist and familiar with working on people's feet, this will feel entirely natural to you, but if not you may need to practise a couple of times with friends and family before it feels comfortable.

It involves simply placing the sole of the patient's foot against the heart of the carer. It doesn't sound much, but it's an act of extreme trust for both and sets up a rapport and intimacy between the two, even more so if the patient's sole touches the carer's heart with bare skin.

If the idea of flesh-to-flesh contact is too daunting (and for some people it's just too intrusive) the foot can be wrapped in silk, or clothed in soft socks and the feet positioned on a cushion.

However it is undertaken, this simple exercise really helps to connect with someone and convey the sense of care that you will be working with.

If we can reach out to others — both from the heart and to the heart — our work comes with a heightened connection and enhanced qualities of love and compassion.

No amount of clever gestures and medical terminology can replace the therapeutic power of working heart-to-heart with someone who is close to the end. Most human beings relax when they are touched, and invisible barriers and unspoken fears melt away.

The Dark Night of the Soul

Jesus appealed to God when he was dying on the cross with heart-breaking vulnerability and rejection, saying 'My God, my God, why has Thou forsaken me?' His words are often echoed by people experiencing 'The Dark Night of the Soul'.

This is a stage when even the most spiritual people temporarily lose their faith and feel utterly abandoned. Along with their belief systems and inner strengths, they start to doubt everything. This is the very lowest point in the pre-death stage, and can last for days (but not usually any longer).

As a soul companion we can really lend our strength to someone going through this episode, which is, I feel, linked to making a final act of surrender, making the decision to let go and trust in whatever must be. I have noticed that it's often experienced in a much deeper way in people who have had very strong religious or spiritual beliefs, and it especially seems to affect priests and healers.

It's as if, for a defined period near the point of death, they must detach from all comforting belief systems and their direct connection with the divine. It's an utterly desolate experience, empty, bleak and a huge chasm to sink into.

For us as carers it's helpful to know that it's just part of the process — another sign that the ego is dissolving and finally realizing that the truth and key to immortality are contained within ourselves. When this is finally accepted and when this surrender has taken place, the energy shifts from fear to enlightenment and can feel like the sun appearing from behind the clouds.

Death or Soul Midwives

Death midwives act as spiritual and energetic guides for those at the time of their death. Forging a deep and intimate bond with the one dying, the midwife supports and assists her charge from across the bridge from this life into a new life on the other shore.

Joellyn St Pierre

HOW SOUL MIDWIVES WORK

'When I am sitting with someone who has probably only hours to live, I'm there to support them in any way that they need. I'm the calm in the middle of the storm,' explains soul midwife, Jo Spiers:

I don't think that you choose to do this sort of work ... it chooses you. I'm still profoundly moved by every death I witness — I'm there to help them experience what it is that they need and I aim to be completely non-judgemental, responsive, compassionate, and very connected to whatever is unfolding.

Jo works as an independent soul midwife in London, having switched to an holistic role after 20 years as a Macmillan nurse. She's helped more than 30 people through the dying process, using the Hospice of the Heart's Gentle Dying method, pioneered by me.

She usually meets for the first time and then begins working with a patient three weeks or so before the death. She's there for the active dying phase (two or three days before death) and often, but not always, right up until the death occurs.

As well as forging very strong ties with her patients, she also talks to them and their families about what is likely to happen, and what choices can be made. After this she establishes how she'll be working with them and also the level of support they'll require, and for how long.

She also works in conjunction with the medical team, complementing their treatment and care.

She doesn't perform any medical procedures, although technically she could because of her previous medical training, but tends the body and soul, ensuring that any death under her care will be as dignified and compassionately supported as possible.

Most midwives visit the family again a few weeks afterwards to discuss any outstanding problems — and bring events to a close. Sometimes they will also facilitate a short ceremony, or have a cup of tea, light a candle, say a prayer and share memories about the person who has died. Jo embraces a multi-faith view and is also a celebrant, which means she can create services or rituals and honours the belief systems of all who come to her.

Extracts from Jo's work journal describe the breadth of her work:

First Visit

Today I met Penelope, who is dying from lung cancer. She's very gregarious and vivacious and surrounded by an adoring and very supportive family. Having been an artist and psychotherapist for 25 years, she tells me that she has been working on personal and spiritual aspects of her death and spirituality for more than 15 years and feels very well-prepared for whatever comes.

I jot it down. But one of the first lessons I've learned is not to assume anything. It's useful that's she's used to talking openly and describing her feelings with strangers. This will take us a long way. But, from working with so many other people, I know that most of us have anxieties and unresolved issues somewhere ... and dying is when they usually surface. We chat and I offer to massage her back, which is aching, with essential oils so that she gets used to my touch.

Second Visit

Penny (as she says she'd like to be known) is in floods of tears. Says her life has gone to pieces since the diagnosis. All her strength has vanished both physically and mentally. She doesn't even think she believes in God any more, everything has let her down (classic dark night of the soul). Am I dying?... Do you know anything about this? She asks all this furiously and really challenges me (this is strange, as I know that she's in the full picture about her prognosis. I've talked openly with her and her husband Peter about her illness and dying). I guess she's feeling denial and fear, which is so common in people who just don't feel that they are ready to go. She hasn't accepted the situation on all levels and appears to be blocking reality. During another massage, we talk about what dying actually is ... and also what it means and feels like to her ... gently and very slowly, we begin to unpack the anxious feelings.

I listen and watch very carefully, noticing just where she stumbles for the right word or holds back because something has flooded her emotions. Her language gives me so many clues as to how she may be feeling and what she is finding difficult to express. She says, 'It's as if a dark shadow is hovering over me, trying to blot out the light of the sun.' I sit quietly beside her, holding her hand and reflecting back to her some of her own thoughts, coaxing her into discovering what she thinks might be the truth and hoping that, by doing this, I'm helping her to find her own strength.

I cut her toenails while she looks at my crystals — and she chooses a heart-shaped rose quartz stone to keep by her bed.

Third Visit

Penny is very bright and also very bossy today. She says she's feeling much better now and can't think what all the tears were about. She says she's been thinking that she wants to do a lot more to help the people she loves before she goes! This entails her giving them some therapy as they come to visit her and telling them things that she knows will help them to heal their own difficult relationships. This is very strengthening to her and partly to do with needing to feel strong, useful and empowered again.

She is very strong and matriarchal and I often get a sense of her teaching me. Every now and then she looks at me and laughs and suggests I try another tack, because I haven't got it quite right. I love this huge generosity and grace on her part.

We laugh a lot together and are already becoming very close.
She asks me to work on her death plan with her and we make
up a visualization about her stepping into a boat as she dies.
At the moment, as we talk, she says she can see it tied up
against a jetty, but it's a long way away and she has to go
underneath a very powerful waterfall before she can reach it.
She asks if I'll give her some hands-on healing. In contrast to
her feisty outer persona, her energy feels very fearful, jangling
and physically weak as I place my hands on her forehead. She
asks me if I can give her a 'top-up' of extra healing energy so
that she can enjoy herself with her visitors this weekend.
Unexpectedly, after the healing session, with her eyes closed,
she holds my hand and tells me about her deepest worries. It's
like a boil being lanced. Lots of tears, then more smiles.

Fourth Visit
I give her healing as requested, as she is feeling very weak.
I do it very carefully so as not to over-stimulate her. Her energy
feels low but stable. As I place my hands on her I sense a
team of angels or higher beings who are working with us.
They introduce themselves to me while I am doing the healing
and suggest that we work together as a team. Guides often

appear when I am giving healing. I don't always mention this to the patient, unless it feels appropriate, but today Penny has somehow sensed that this has happened. She wonders who it is who's come forward to help her. Before I offer any suggestions, she says, 'You'll think I'm nuts, but I think it's Jesus. He told me to relax and told me to give him my fears and he'd sort them out.' We both laugh, but with a hint of seriousness.

Fifth Visit

Next day Peter opens the door, beaming and radiant. He says the healing has made a huge difference. Penny is so much better, stronger, happier, calmer — she's even been down for lunch of cheese on toast...

Upstairs, Penny's lying on her bed looking very serene. She says there's been a miracle, she's shifted and she feels 'herself' again, and is not afraid of dying any more

I used my Tingshaws (small Tibetan cymbals) in the corners of the room ... to clear away the stagnant energy (she's been in bed for three weeks now)... and although getting very weak, she asks if we can work with sound. I used my broken heart-chakra singing bowl, sensing some grief held within her that might need to be cleared, before starting the healing.

Did 20 minutes of that and felt huge surges of energy in the room. Then spent ten minutes on her feet (ice-cold)... and put lots of warm healing energy into them, I wrapped them up and swaddled them (big smile from Penny).

She said she been holding the little heart stone I'd given to her all night as she slept and found it very comforting when her breathing was bad.

At the end of the visit she said she felt 'safe again' and asked please could I come again tomorrow. She thought she'd like to go downstairs again tonight ... but wondered if she would have enough energy to do it.

Sixth Visit

Penny feeling very breathless and scared. She's dying ... She's feeling anxious about something, which is lurking. It's big and black and horrendous ... and she thinks it might be to do with her sister with whom she fell out many years ago. She says she 'really hates' her and is scared that this 'woman' will waltz into the room and try to take over at the end. We work out a practical strategy for dealing with this, involving various friends and neighbours who will be on standby.

I give healing to the bad lung (seeing with my third eye which one it is). I sense it's black and spidery in the middle, with thin tendrils coming out of it. I try to remove it by dissolving it with a blast of golden light. Then I give the good lung a spring-clean and try to energize it to work better. Then we work on some breathing techniques, bringing the breath right down into the stomach via the healthy lung.

Together we imagine a blue light coming in with the in-breath and making a clear channel into the lung. We sit for ages just breathing in and out. She asks me to wait while she goes to the loo because she's scared that she'll be breathless afterwards. She is, but we coax the breath back to normal by practising the breathing exercises we learned a few days ago ... Afterwards, while she is resting, she thanks me for everything I have done and says she'll never forget me. She asks me if I'll carry her to her boat very soon, and swim alongside it for a while until it reaches the shore across the water. I promise I will. Two days later Penny died. She'd asked for healing, anointing and singing bowls to be used as she lost consciousness and up until the time she stopped breathing. She passed away early in the morning, making a long peaceful-sounding out-breath, with her family sitting around her.

Soul Midwives and Psychopomps

Soul midwives are steadily growing in number —
working in towns, cities and communities across
the world. Many of them have dual occupations
as therapist-counsellors, mediums, psychics,
healers and shamen, and through their work they
are helping many people have a more enlightened
attitude to death.

Some are even extending their services and acting
as modern-day psychopomps — the ancient name
given to those who guided the souls of mortals
after death. Hermes, Archangel St Michael, the
Inuit goddess Pinga, St Brigit, Hecate and Thoth
were all believed to work with the dying and dead
in this way.

This is a very specialized and esoteric role which
is re-emerging at this very significant time in the
planet's history.

Many people who die are not even conscious that they are dead. They pass without even being aware of what has happened. As a result, the layers of 'stuck' souls are stacking up on the earth's etheric mantle.

There can be many reasons for this. Sometimes, because there is a great attachment to loved ones, partners, children or even pets. A very strong link to a physical location or object — such as homes, cars, possessions — may also hold them back. And, occasionally, addictions — such as to alcohol, drugs, sex or gambling — can distort the delicate balance of the psyche, making transition an impossible wrench because the soul cannot tear itself away from the source of the addiction.

There is also a general soul malaise, a symptom of our modern times which is caused by spiritual disconnection. Sadly we live in a spiritually bankrupt age, which makes dying harder than it needs to be.

An honouring of the importance of the sacred and the divine in all aspects of our lives has very low priority in our world today.

To release without attachment, you have to have trust and be ready to move on — but also realize that you have your own free will. This isn't to paint too gloomy a picture — we are never completely abandoned by the loving wise ones who wait for us patiently on the other side. Those who are unable, for whatever reason, to embrace the essential journey of their soul, may linger in a twilight world and in a state of neutral suspension for some time, but they will eventually be, as we all will be, encouraged to walk towards the light.

The tsunami in 2004 resulted in a massive, sudden surge of transiting souls, many of whom found it difficult to sever their connection with their earthly bodies. The harrowing events when the World Trade Center towers collapsed in New York in 2001 had a similar impact. Teams of soul midwives, light-workers and shamen are working still to relieve this collective soul trauma by escorting souls back home.

This global view has been channelled and confirmed by sensitives working separately and in distant places throughout the world. The men and women serving the spiritual health of their peoples, separated by different languages and spanning entire continents, all describe the same scenario.

CHAPTER THREE

Preparing for the Great Journey

Death is not extinguishing the light; it is putting out the lamp because dawn has come.

Rabindranath Tagore

Death Journey Work

When I am asked to help someone who is dying, we start straight away to work on a plan which will take them towards their death ... and sometimes beyond. This plan, although very flexible, will act as a map to keep us on track.

We begin by exploring what sort of death they would like and then work out how this can be achieved.

Besides the spiritual aspects, there are lots of practicalities to address, such as where the death is likely to occur, whether or not they have a living will, whom would they like to be with them at the end (and whom not), whether or not they belong to an organized Church or require any important rituals (such as last rites), and whether there are any unresolved relationship issues, specific worries or fears to be worked with.

Gradually a picture builds as to how best to help them. The plan becomes an intimate contract between us.

Another very important aspect of this planning, or Journey Work, is also about helping people to find their own inner strengths and resources, and showing them how to work with their own free will to help them through the dark and lonely phases. One of the ways in which we can do this is by harnessing the power of their own imagination and creating a series of visual and narrative ideas. This becomes a source of specific images and sensations that will help them find calm and safety whenever they need it.

For instance, the journey often starts with a visualization — it might be a walk up a steep and winding path towards a mountain, or on a boat floating down a river, or walking down steps leading into a beautiful garden.

We may also choose a piece of music, or several pieces that are significant and meaningful in some way and can be played to accompany the visualization or help with relaxation.

We will also imagine a healing sanctuary where they will go to rest and recover after death, imagining just what it will look like and who will be there waiting for them to help with their care (often a parent, child, best friend, former pet or a holy figure).

Sometimes, if the person has a spiritual guide or guru, we invoke or meet them in a meditation and ask them if they will be involved with us in the Journey Work.

Many people like to 'power up' a talisman for their journey (a significant ring or stone, or any possession that brings a feeling of protection with it).

All these ideas are expanded and developed over the weeks or days while we work together, and may also include drawing, writing and keeping a dream journal.

Making a Good Death Plan

If someone has asked you to help them plan their death and help them once they are too weak or ill to put their plans into place, this is what you'll need to discuss:

- *Where would you like to die? At home, in hospital or a hospice?*

- *How much information would you like to be given?*

- *What level of pain-relief would you require?*

- *Do you want to remain lucid at all times and able to make decisions?*

- *Would you prefer the information to be given to a proxy (i.e. a partner or relative)?*

- *Would you like any religious ceremonies or rituals prior to death?*

- *Singing, chanting or poems to be spoken aloud.*

- *Would you like to be anointed or receive healing?*

- *Would you like your holistic therapies continued when you are close to death?*

- *Whom would you like to have (or not have) with you?*

- *Are there any outstanding issues (relationships, emotional, financial) to be resolved?*

- *How long would you like to be left after you have died before you are removed and prepared for burial or cremation?*

Breath

We are born on a breath and we die on a breath. All that separates us from the next life and this one is ... one small breath.

Breathing difficulties, and the panic that this can cause, can be one of the most distressing aspects of dying, but it's a problem that we can really help with.

When we are frightened or worried we instinctively take quicker and more rapid breaths which make us tense up, increasing our fear.

Simple breathing techniques are easy to both use and learn and can really make a difference to someone who is panicking when they can't get enough breath to fill their lungs. These exercises can also calm down an anxious carer and are useful to learn at the beginning. I often commence and end a session with a period of mindful breathing. It calms everything down and helps bring any issues into focus that may need working on during the session.

Imagine that you are a conductor (of breath rather than music) and that you are trying to synchronize a passage of music that's lost its rhythm.

You'll need to sit for a few minutes to concentrate on your companion's breathing, tuning in to the rise and fall of their chest.

Then, start mirroring and copying their breathing pattern, making an 'Ahh' sound on the out-breath.

Gradually, after five or six breaths, extend the out-breath to a longer 'Aaaaaaaaaaahhhhhhh'. Encourage them to make this sound with you, if they are able to, for at least ten breaths until they feel calm and safe.

If you are feeling agile and the person dying isn't connected to too many tubes and machinery, you can get into bed with them, cradling them from behind and encouraging them to lean back onto you. As they relax, supported by your body, they will instinctively start to feel the rhythm of your breathing and heartbeat and instinctively interact with it, becoming centred and more peaceful.

The Senses

We take them so much for granted, but the senses are truly the gateways to the soul. Through the portals of hearing, seeing, touching, tasting and smelling we are able to interpret our experience of the world and awaken the universal imagination that co-creates our own personal stories.

Throughout our lives, body and soul are inextricably woven together. But during our dying time the links that connect them are gradually loosened so that they can separate and eventually detach. To enable this to happen, the senses alter the way in which they work, very subtly, evolving to our changing needs. As this happens, new and different information surfaces, enabling us to face the final changes that we need to experience towards the end of life. This expanded sense of time and reality re-orientates us as our consciousness changes.

Dying people are very delicate and fragile, and this is partly because their senses are unusually heightened. They are vulnerable to extremes such as bright lights, loud noises, and especially uncomfortable surroundings.

As their 'vision' changes, they sometimes appear to see things that we cannot see. Their hearing may also become so highly sensitized that they will hear things that we cannot hear. Their sense of taste may also change and they may crave unusual foods, just as pregnant women do.

Around the time of death, our senses seem to work to bring us back into step with our inner needs and, as they morph, they trigger shifts in perception and release psychological blockages which may be hampering part of the dying process.

This is why working with sound, touch and smell is so productive and enriching at the end of life.

HEARING

Hearing is the final sense that we lose. Even if someone appears to be deeply asleep, sedated, unconscious or in a coma and all signs of life appear to be fading, remember that they can still probably hear you and understand what you are saying.

Hearing is also our most dynamic faculty. It's totally developed at birth, unlike sight and smell, and it penetrates our deepest being, inspiring our connection with the outer world.

Many of us have lost the instinct to reach inside ourselves and enjoy silence. Indeed, it is the still centre within all of us that is needed for the inner reflective work that nourishes the soul. We constantly fill our space with loud discordant noise, televisions, radios, iPods, telephones, without opening happily into silence. For some people, of course, silence equals nothingness and can be very threatening. But sometimes, just sitting with someone in companionable silence can be healing and may help them to turn inwards and access their well of inner peace.

Ears are shaped like question marks, their labyrinthine chambers burrow beneath our skull and are placed close-up to the brain, making direct contact with the source of our thinking.

If you are sitting with someone who is dying, or seriously ill, avoid difficult or jarring conversations. Discourage visitors from having antagonistic conversations (one poor woman lay dying as her quarrelling relatives sat on either side of the bed squabbling about who'd inherit the new plasma television).

The caress of the voice is soothing and intimate, and words have great power. Speak kindly, gently, softly and tell them what you are doing, or who is coming to visit them today. If you have to leave the room, to go for a meal or to make a telephone call (even if it's only for five minutes), let them know.

A lot of people are worried that that they won't know what to say to someone who is dying — they don't want to make matters worse by saying the wrong thing.

What Sort of Things Do Dying People Like to Hear?

I think, very importantly, to know that they are loved and have been loved and that their lives have had meaning. Even a tramp sleeping rough on the streets will have been loved by a mother, sibling, partner or someone or -thing (perhaps a dog, or the birds they have fed in the park) who has had contact with them.

You can extend this, if you know the person well, by reciting happy moments back to them: childhood memories, meeting a loved one for the first time, the birth of their children, happy holidays, etc.

Many people like to be reassured that their loved ones and pets have been taken care of and that their houses are being watched over. Also that their friends are sending their love and thoughts.

When you speak, be sure to use the name that is their own (not Mr or Mrs, or Nan, or Uncle) but their full name or nickname they were given by their parents, or the one that they have used for most of their life.

Hearing your own name spoken to you can be very intimate. Our names carry a specific energy, our unique essence and, with them, a sense of belonging. According to tribal teachings, we each have a spirit name from the moment we first come into existence, and the name follows us from life to life, and back into the spirit world afterwards, and throughout our lifetime we will be given clues and reminders as to what it is. When we die, perhaps we remember our true names once again.

SMELL

Just smelling a rose, a freshly peeled orange or a baked cake can shift our mood dramatically, making us happy one moment or reflective and peaceful the next.

Our smell sensors are connected to the limbic system, which scientists say is the most ancient and primitive part of our brains, and also thought to be the seat of emotion.

Many clinical studies into the therapeutic use of smell have proved that certain aromas can enhance the efficacy of medicine-based pain relief as well as making people feel more positive. Experiments have also shown that scents entering the left nostril are more likely to be perceived as positive while those breathed in through the right nostril are negative. This is worth remembering if you are wondering where to position an oil burner, or on which side of the pillow to place a handkerchief scented with essential oils.

Sensitivity to smell declines with advancing age and also as the result of certain illnesses, but when we are well we are able to differentiate between 4,000 and 10,000 different aromas.

Scents also have the power to trigger memory — eucalyptus is strong and clean and reminiscent of childhood vapour rubs, the sharp notes of pine are purifying and antiseptic, lavender and rose are soothing, but vanilla is the most universally accepted comfort smell, perhaps because it reminds people of the nurturing warmth of mother's milk. In a UK trial involving cancer patients undergoing stressful chemotherapy and radiotherapy treatments, the wafting scent of vanilla led to a 63 per cent reduction in anxiety symptoms.

And in the old days, onions were peeled to help people suffering from laboured breathing — perhaps the smell triggered an opening of the airways. It's an old trick and certainly worth trying.

There are many ways that we can use smell to help the dying:

- *essential oils in burners, diffusers or in sprays (see section on oils, pages 170–2)*

- *scented soaps and creams*

- *washing bed linen with rose or lavender water*

- *spritzing the air with scented floral waters*

- *scented candles*

- *burning incense.*

Dying is an opportunity to uncover what is hidden. To see the sacred is to gradually remove the obscurations, the perceptions that block our capacity to recognize the truth of what was always present. Dying is at its heart a sacred act, it is itself a time, a space and a process of surrender and transformation.

Frank Ostaeski, founder of the Zen Hospice project

SEEING

When people are dying, their peripheral field of vision narrows and they are only able to focus on what's straight ahead. When you come to visit them it will help if you stand at the bottom of their bed to introduce yourself (even if they know who you are) before sitting beside them.

Our sight is, of course, also symbolic and connected to our inner vision of things. Dying people often appear to use their eyes and sight for seeing beyond our reality and for peering into their inner deeper world.

As mentioned, all the senses sharpen and intensify before death. Dying people often say that they can see things that we cannot see, such as dancing lights, colours, friends and pets who have already passed on.

I was asked to keep an elderly woman called Marjory company at the hospice for an hour or so one evening. She was in her eighties and close to death, but still had a deep craving for company and liked chatting whenever she was awake. She'd suddenly fall asleep in mid-sentence, which made attempts to converse frustrating and labour-intensive, and the busy nurses just didn't have the time to sit and be with her as much as she would have liked.

While we sat, she told me that her father visited her every night at eight to 'tuck me up and put me to bed'. She asked me if I would stay on to meet him. She dozed on and off and I busied myself nearby doing other jobs around the ward.

When I looked in on her at 7.55 she was fast asleep and snoring, so I started to put on my coat to go home. But on the dot of eight, while I hovered in the doorway, she suddenly opened her eyes and glowed with immense pleasure, looking like a sixteen-year-old in a rapture.

Completely oblivious of anyone being in the room with her, she giggled and chatted to the blank space ahead, as if in a hypnotized state. I couldn't see or sense anything but I knew that beyond doubt her father had come to 'see' her and safely settle her for the night.

TOUCH

I sat with Emily (78) a couple of days before she died. She'd been in and out of consciousness but was awake now and able to take small sips of water. She didn't want to talk much and was very withdrawn. She'd been complaining of pain in her foot, so I asked if she'd like me to rub some cream on it for her. She nodded and rested her foot on my lap. After massaging her sole for about 15 minutes I sensed her mood change; she seemed to soften and relax. With tears rolling down her cheeks she told me that that she'd been widowed for 40 years and no one had properly touched her since.

Touch heals in a direct link from the heart and the hands — it's a natural form of communication without words, and as well as being reassuring it brings a powerful sense of presence.

It can be as minimal as just looking into someone's eyes — the person you are caring for will know that you are willing to sit with them, hold their hand and treat them with respect and dignity. You may be anxious or hesitant about touching someone that you don't know very well, but don't worry, your heart will guide your hands.

Sadly, many dying and seriously ill people are only touched as part of a medical examination or procedure. And if they are suffering from a contagious disease such as MRSA, or have an illness that makes them smell unpleasant, many of them become virtually untouchable. They can quickly feel very isolated and alone.

Conventional massage isn't appropriate to use on people as they are dying — it's too strong and invasive — but there are many other gentle ways of touching such as a soft back or shoulder rub, a butterfly kiss on the hand and, if even that's too hard to bear, a soft blow of breath against the skin or the waft of a downy feather.

All forms of loving touch can bring comforting feelings and often unlock emotions that have been unexpressed for years.

Many soul midwives also practise therapeutic touch, a form of traditional hands-on healing — either directly on the body or with their hands placed four or five inches away in the aura of the person.

Anyone can use touch for healing as long as they have love in their hearts. Occasionally, though, I have come across people who aren't comfortable with being touched in any way. Because of this, be very sensitive, as the person may not be able to tell you this, if they are past speaking, but may only be able to convey their discomfort by tensing up or looking distressed. Never inflict your wish to comfort on someone if they don't look as if they are comfortable with what you're doing.

One of the easiest ways to start is by offering a very simple hand massage with scented oils or creams ... Feet are also wonderful, although not pleasant for everyone, as they might feel ticklish. Washing someone's feet is a very nurturing and humbling act.

Healing

People often go into such a deep space during a healing session that everything worrying them leaves them for a short while — this experience results in people feeling much calmer and able to find a safe and peaceful place within themselves.

Reiki

Reiki means 'universal life-force energy' and the system is a powerful form of touch therapy originating from Japan. By channelling the energy around someone, you can treat them on a physical and emotional level simultaneously.

When people are feeling very distraught, they often feel a restored sense of balance following a treatment, as if they've been given a glimpse of the 'whole' picture.

They may still be feeling a huge sense of loss but they can begin to move into the process of letting go after a session of healing or Reiki.

Colour

> Whenever Christine wore her green nightie, we noticed that she'd become tetchy and anxious. She'd been suffering from Alzheimer's for over five years and was increasingly hard to communicate with. But when we put her into an identical pink nightie she'd immediately become somehow softer and happier. You can guess which nightie we rushed to get washed and dried.
>
> Judith, a care assistant

Colours, like smells and sound, can have a great influence on our moods and emotions. When used therapeutically they can also enhance the effects of other forms of healing.

Some colours will soothe, some will stimulate, others inspire. The colours we choose when we are working with the dying can have a profound effect, as they connect with so many esoteric aspects of our psyche — particularly our chakra system.

Chakras

The chakras are centres of energy within the body and store the vital life force described in Eastern medicine as *prana, Chi* or *Ki*. Although the chakras are invisible, you can sometimes sense them as swirling wheels of coloured energy. There are seven main chakras in the body, sited between the base of the spine and the top of the head:

1st chakra: Root

2nd chakra: Sacral

3rd chakra: Solar Plexus

4th chakra: Heart

5th chakra: Throat

6th chakra: Brow

7th chakra: Crown.

When we die, the chakras open wide. Some therapists use coloured light torches which focus a beam of coloured light onto an acupressure point or chakra to help clear energy blockages. Soul midwives often use coloured silk squares draped onto parts of the body to bring a sense of calm and security during treatments.

- *Red — encourages adrenaline and can be positive for empowerment, positivity and focus in early active stages of illness. Too strong for the final stages unless the person actually requests it.*

- *Orange — appetite-stimulant, friendly, outgoing, stimulating.*

- *Yellow — very cheerful and sociable, useful for alleviating depression. Warm and optimistic.*

- *Green — the colour of balance and harmony, relaxing, connecting with nature.*

- *Pink — feminine, heart energy, love, nurturing, softness.*

- *Blue — peaceful, calming, stabilizing, has been shown to reduce blood pressure and respiration and heart rate. Balancing and comforting.*

- *Purple — the highest frequency in the colour spectrum. Connects people with their spirituality.*

- *White — clean, simple and crisp, yet too sterile for some. It's a very good background for using with other colours.*

How Does It Feel to Die?

It can really help us to help the dying if we can understand what they might be feeling or experiencing. Many people have described what it feels like, and this is backed up by descriptions in ancient texts.

When we die, our soul leaves our physical body. Most of us experience this in a smooth and seamless way, shifting from one plane of existence to another. As we move out of the body we are able to look down and see our empty 'shell'. We then enter a tunnel of light where we are greeted by friends or spiritual beings, and are enveloped in the purest energy of love.

Before this happens we feel:

- a chill spreading up through the chakras

- a tugging sensation as the subtle bodies detach

- a sensation of rocking backwards and forwards

- *snapping and tearing sounds as physical and subtle bodies part*

- *disorientation (not being sure where sounds etc. are coming from)*

- *altered sense of time*

- *senses stop working, starting with touch*

- *taste and smell go at same time*

- *sight and hearing are the last to go*

- *loud buzzing noises are heard*

- *bright lights or a tunnel leading towards light appears.*

Working in the Dream State

The Dream State is the place we inhabit when we leave our bodies at night and expand into the astral realms. When we are dying we spend more and more time there, especially when we are experimenting with how it feels to be out of our bodies.

Shamen shift their consciousness in order to merge with the souls of others. They use this deep level of connection to help them meet totem animals and guides when they perform soul retrieval and ancestral work.

Soul midwives sometimes enter this inner space of the person they're working with to work with the dying when they are unconscious or out of their bodies for long periods.

Many healers and sensitives also instinctively do this by temporarily tuning in to the interior space of the people they are helping. The Dream State is the numinous, timeless realm that we visit when we sleep. It's where our spirit and soul expand and reconnect with our true and eternal aspects.

Working in the Dream State is a very specialized form of healing requiring years of practice and mentoring by someone already very experienced in this field.

It can be overwhelming both for the healer and the person receiving healing, as it can tip both off-balance by exposing them to the powerful energies of the inner realms of the psyche, a bit like the effects of psychedelic drugs.

As one soul midwife I have worked with said, 'Working in this state is like white-water swimming, if you are still using arm bands — there's an adrenaline rush and it's amazing, but the waters can be very choppy and once or twice I thought I'd go under.'

However, being invited into someone's inner space during tough times can and does have its place when we are helping someone to die gently.

Michael, a young actor nursing his partner Peter during his final illness, says that when Peter was unconscious or deeply asleep following treatment, it was as if an invisible, energetic window flew open. They could be closer and share their love on a profoundly deeper level.

Although Peter wasn't up to having long conversations physically, it was if they were carrying on an intense conversation by telepathy.

This is connecting to the Dream State in its simplest form. If you are caring for someone you are very close to — a parent, partner or child — these deep inner levels often easily and spontaneously open up and invite us to enter.

It is always a sacred honour to enter anyone's inner sanctum, as it's where they are laid bare with no shell of protection. Because of this, the intimacy and trust involved must never be violated. There are some clear rules for entering this space, even if we know and love the person very well.

We must always ask for permission to enter, each and every time. If they are unconscious we need to go into a state of prayer or meditation to ask permission. Sometimes, despite having done this work with someone many times before, you may suddenly be told 'No!'

If this happens, withdraw with respect and love and know that the time is not right for this work, for whatever reason. It does not necessarily mean that you will be barred from entering again, but just that on this occasion it is inappropriate for the 'wider good'.

It's as if we hold that person's beating heart in our hands when we work on the deep and inner levels. It is incredibly tender, and we must handle it with exquisite grace, and be totally responsible for its safekeeping.

Sometimes I sense I am barred because I am too tired or not being mindful enough to concentrate. At other times it's as if the person is involved in 'other' work when I attempt to be there, and I'm politely told that the time isn't right — a bit like when you visit someone in hospital and there are curtains around the bed.

ENTERING THE DREAM STATE

First centre yourself, surround yourself with a protective cloak of golden light (or whatever protection visualization best works for you), concentrate on your breathing and reach a deep state of calm and awareness. Call on your own guides to stand with you, and invite the guides of your friend also to be involved for the highest good.

Imagine the soul of your friend and reach out to make a connection with it. You may perceive it as a beating rhythm, or note, a glowing light or colour, or perhaps none of these. But when you have found it, ask silently if it is appropriate for you to be working with them. If the answer is yes, then slowly merge into it.

When you are secure and comfortable you might want to ask:

- Are you in pain?

- Is there anything worrying you that I can help with?

- Would you like some healing?

- Is there anything I can be doing for you?

When you leave the Dream State, withdraw gently and spend a little time alone, in silence, to re-orientate yourself.

Ten Very Simple Tips If You Are Sitting with a Friend Who Is Dying

1. Touch can be very healing. Gentle hand-holding or stroking of the hands and arms are gestures we instinctively use to comfort. A very simple hand massage using scented oils or creams can be a great way of communicating with someone when words are hard to find.

2. Moisten a dying person's lips and eyes regularly with warm damp cotton wool or sponge mouth-wipes. Use mouthwashes (cinnamon tincture in tepid water is very good, as commercial brands may taste too strong) if your friend is finding it too strenuous or uncomfortable to brush their teeth.

3. Check that their ears are lying flat and comfortable on the pillow and are not

squashed, as this can lead to circulation problems and severe discomfort.

4. If you are able to, change the position of their head and shoulders every hour.

5. Learn and share some very simple breathing techniques (similar to the ones that pregnant women use during labour). They can be very soothing and can help bring calm after anxious moments.

6. Learn a simple visualization technique which you can use as you sit and keep your friend company. This can be a useful distraction while you are waiting for pain relief to become effective.

7. Burn essential oils in a burner in the bedroom. Lavender, rose, geranium, lemon or myrtle all smell lovely, and besides scenting the air they will revive and restore the spirits of

everyone who comes into the room. In India, sandalwood is often used to help the spirit depart from the body.

8. If your friend has to be cared for away from home, in hospital or a care home, take their own pillows, duvet or bed covers for extra comfort. A present of a soft goose-down pillow may also be really appreciated.

9. Softly singing and whispering gentle assurances that 'all is well and all will be well' or similar phrases can be very soothing.

10. Switch off harsh lighting. Candlelight is preferable (but not in a room where oxygen is being used), but if this isn't practical a side light with a soft low-watt orange bulb is kinder to dying eyes.

We got a baby alarm when George was dying, which was switched on day and night. He liked it because it meant we could get on with things downstairs and he didn't have to get out of bed or shout to get us to hear him.

Alice

Vigiling

All around the world, communities have their traditional way of keeping vigil, sitting and keeping watch over those who are dying.

In Africa they tell stories about the ancestors so that the dying person will find their way back to them; in India they chant holy mantras and anoint the person with precious oils; in Iceland they sit around the communal fire and gather in guardian spirits.

The Celtic shaman, writer and singer Caitlin Matthews tells of women 'keeping watch' on the western isles of Scotland, who sing the eerie and sonorous song of the native red shank bird to steer the soul home: 'Tweeet... tweeet... tweet... peelee... peelee woooooooooo' and the dying person's name is repeated and sung, intertwined with the dipping soaring notes of the bird to aid the soul's release.

Six thousand miles away in Tibet, when a death is imminent, gleaming brass singing bowls or temple bells are stroked with a wooden mallet until the sound throbs and fills the room in a column of energy to honour the death.

Singing, praying, listening and watching, both as a family or including the wider community, are all ways of sitting ... in vigil.

As Irish poet and philosopher John O'Donohue explains, 'A blessing is a circle of light drawn around a person to protect, heal and strengthen' — this is just the sense of caring guardianship that vigiling invokes.

Sadly, many of us have forgotten just how to do this now, especially if we are sitting with someone dying away from home, in a hospital or care home, and we may feel stupid or that we are getting in the way somehow. But wherever you are and whomever you are with, vigiling is one of the most devotional acts of loving care that you can offer.

Shauna Ray, a former Macmillan nurse who now works as a soul midwife, gives families ideas on how they may want to create their vigil with their dying ones:

We need to honour the dying experience and nurture it by paying it full attention, kindness and love, emptying our minds and really concentrating on what is unfolding. As we do this, we naturally become softer, more compassionate, peaceful, loving and kinder and able to really reach out to the person who is dying with an open and loving heart. Intimacy is sacred — a secret trust — a soulful commitment. Don't go in with your own baggage, just observe the mystery of the other person. People ask me if I experience fear or sorrow while I work — none of that manifests when I'm with the dying person. It's their time, not mine. Any burden or sorrow or wounds of your own disappear. You hold the person and keep vigil while they quietly, almost invisibly, shimmer an indescribable membrane of light.

VIGILING TIPS

- *Sitting together*

- *Sharing silence*

- *Talking or listening*

- *Reading inspirational texts*

- *Singing or chanting*

- *Healing touch*

- *Invoking Blessings*

*There is a light that shines beyond all things on earth,
Beyond us all,*

Beyond the heavens,

Beyond the highest heavens.

This is the light that shines in our hearts.

Chandogya Upanishad

CHAPTER FOUR
The Soul

The soul, like death, is a great mystery to us. But the more I work with people who are dying and see with my own eyes the profound spiritual shifts that happen at this time, the more in awe of the soul and its enigmatic ways I become.

You will probably have your own ideas about what happens to us after we die, and also whether or not the idea of the soul is important or even relevant to you.

But even conventional science acknowledges the idea that we are more than just our physical bodies — the first law of thermodynamics states that energy cannot be created or destroyed.

Water can be solid, liquid, vapour or even invisible (steam and super-steam) and no one doubts that it continues to exist. As we are also energetic beings, why should we be any different? It makes sense to me that we, too, must continue to exist on some level after death.

The existence of the soul, just like God, is of course impossible to prove. A survey conducted by Ipsos Mori in 2007 revealed that 54 per cent of all men and 69 per cent of women in the UK believe that we have souls, and that 47 per cent of all people polled believed in life after death.

Ideas about the soul seem to share the same slot in people's minds as angels, ghosts, fairies and other unworldly beings and apparitions. They often regard soul issues as too deep, too superstitious, spooky or downright weird. Not many families sit around talking about their souls as they eat their supper.

Yet the soul seems to surface and become most alive when we are dying. It awakens, expands and hungers for recognition in the final days of so many people — often for the first time in their lives.

The journey towards death leads us to the greatest potential for soul growth that we ever encounter. Looking after someone's spiritual needs as they die brings an added edge of expectancy and fulfilment to the caring role.

Watching, listening for and hearing signs that this soul growth is beginning is an extraordinary experience, similar to witnessing the 'quickening' that occurs when a baby begins to stir in the womb (a time recognized by many as the moment when the soul of the baby has entered the body).

In its simplest sense, the soul appears to be — as all the great religions advocate — the part of us that never dies, the spark of divine consciousness that lives in all of us, eternally, linking us back to God.

Some people also perceive the soul as some higher form of themselves — their guardian angel, a personal daimon or another, disconnected, discarnate aspect of themselves.

There's also great confusion between the nature of soul and the nature of spirit. To many people, these are completely interchangeable and one and the same thing.

Having watched the dying and seen the shifts that occur, I feel that the spirit is the transitory and ego-based aspect of our personality relating to who we have been in this lifetime. It is fused to the ego and drives us on, throughout our lives, in an upwards, soaring, expansive and spiralling motion. It finally disperses and vanishes into the air element, dissolving at the point of death.

In contrast to the spirit, I see the soul as our eternal template — a map of everything we are and have the potential to be. It spans all time and eternity. It is the great I AM presence of the mystics, the primordial image of who we are. It's nature is deep, solemn and permanent. It evolves in a downward, labyrinthine and circular movement and embraces all the complex, timeless dynamics of who we are and our relationship to everything around us.

The constant tension between soul and spirit is the load-bearing mechanism of our inner scaffolding. It's the matrix supporting the bricks and mortar of our imagination, intuition and senses, and gives us our potential for both understanding and also becoming who we are.

As the Lord Krishna says in *The Bhagavad Gita*:

The soul or the self cannot be killed, cannot be slain, cannot be drowned, and cannot be burned. It is immortal. Just as a person changes his garments from day to day, so does a person change his body from incarnation to incarnation.

The greatest longing of the soul is the unknown. It thrives on challenge and surrender. Yet most of us are afraid to follow this yearning because it lies outside our vision and our control. Death leads away from all we know, beyond our closest horizon, but our souls know the destination.

Soul Pain

As well as physical pain, most of us are affected by deeper scars, or soul wounds, which don't respond to morphine or sedatives. They exist deep inside, within the dark shadow areas of the psyche, and they hurt when we least expect them to. They hold us back and stop us from opening ourselves fully to the experience of letting go and surrendering. These wounds are usually connected with:

- *abandonment*

- *betrayal*

- *denial*

- *rejection*

- *a fear of not being good enough or of not being loveable.*

As human beings we have a great tendency to run away from suffering, constantly burying our deepest issues. When time is short we can't always help to resolve these soul wounds, but we can look and listen for any unspoken worries and pray for them to be resolved, addressed or cleared on a higher level, beyond our control.

Dying people can be very emotional, angry and often manipulative. This is partly to do with processing their own shadow pain and conflict which they disown and then project onto the world around them. Shadow material can be individual, it can belong to families or it can be collective, such as that belonging to a country or racial group. Sometimes it involves all three levels.

All wounds can make a tear in the soul and, as with fear, working with distressed people can magnify all our own unresolved issues of helplessness, inner pain and grief.

As John O'Donohue says in his book *Anam Cara*:

> When you love someone who is very hurt, one of the worst things you can do is to directly address the hurt and make an issue of it. A strange dynamic comes alive in the soul if you make something into an issue. It becomes a habit and keeps recurring in a pattern. Frequently it is better to simply acknowledge that there is a wound there but then stay away from it. Every chance you get, shine the gentle light of the soul in on the wound.

Recognizing our own soul wounds and confronting them can help us to begin to help others. Compassion is a virtuous skill, but it does mean to 'suffer' with others. To be stronger and more grounded it is better to listen and to be able to help with an attitude of pure love, but with the intention of staying separate. Healthy boundaries should prevent us from entering fully into someone else's pain. As long as we are able to listen and connect deeply with our hearts, we will truly be of service.

By its nature, dying is about ending relationships — our relationship to ourselves, to those we love and for those who care for us. Of course, each individual soul is very different. The wounds we suffer become a lifetime's affliction, yet at death there's a chance to cast them off.

Soul Friends

Having a true soul friend is very warm and comforting at all stages of life, but especially when you are dying.

The Celtic tradition, which is so rich in meaningful rituals to help the dying, has two expressions of soul companions: *Anam Cara* means 'soul friend' and *Anam-Aire* means 'soul carer'.

When we become a soul friend or soul carer to someone, we hold their heart in our hand as tenderly as if it was a fragile egg about to hatch. It is the greatest privilege to help someone to die well and to be there to help them in any way that we can.

A soul friend is a person to whom you can reveal the deepest intimacies of your life, too — your innermost self, mind and heart. A soul carer is someone who guides us with wisdom and knowledge and who has a responsibility for understanding our soul's needs during times of transition for its ultimate and constantly evolving journey.

Intensive compassion or tender loving care is the simplest essence of helping someone to die gently.

HOW TO BE A GOOD SOUL COMPANION

Sitting with someone who is suffering from intense pain without trying to fix or hide it is a harder task than it sounds.

In her book *Waiting for God*, the French philosopher and writer Simone Weil suggests, 'Those who are unhappy have no need for anything else in this world other than people capable of giving them their attention.'

Weil was right. In order to truly help we need to be authentic and be open about our feelings:

- *Meet your friend 'where they are at' rather than where you'd like them to be.*

- *Resist the urge to fix, or rescue, or impose your own beliefs.*

- *Help them find their own source of peace and strength.*

- *Listen and share, but be silent if that's required.*

- *Help them to cultivate a big perspective and see the long view.*

- *Have a non-judgemental attitude — encourage your friend to find and express his or her own meaning of life.*

- *Honour and support their ideas, attitudes and memories.*

- *Offer unconditional love, compassion and confidentiality.*

- *Put yourself in the dying person's place and check your perceptions of their needs with them.*

- *Don't make assumptions.*

- *Cultivate empathy (not pity) — you are equal, not better than them.*

- *Show true compassion and love, and in so doing create an atmosphere of trust and peace that supports and inspires, which at the deepest level helps the dying to heal themselves spiritually.*

CHAPTER FIVE

The Stages of Dying

When we die there is so much more going on than at first meets the eye.

According to Eastern medicine, which has studied death as an exact science for thousands of years, there are four distinct and very separate stages evident in the dying process. These can take place very gradually over a period of months and weeks. Sometimes they merge seamlessly within a space of several hours or, in the case of very sudden death, within minutes.

The Four Primal Elements

These stages, which manifest psycho-spiritually as well as purely physically, are based around the idea that our bodies are composed of the four primal elements: Earth, Water, Fire and, lastly, Air. These elements reflect our inherent vitality, influencing our moods, the ways in which we express ourselves — and even our dreams.

As they withdraw and dissolve they present a set of signs and symptoms which give us very useful clues as to how much life force the person has remaining, and also what he or she is experiencing on an inner level.

They show us how we can best support the dying person as they reach each stage — for example, someone in the Air Stage may benefit from help with their breathing, or from hearing beautiful music to help reduce their anxiety.

Death happens when each of these four elements has withdrawn and the body is reduced to an empty shell.

Although Western medicine has yet to embrace these ideas, more and more doctors and nurses are beginning to recognize these subtle signs and use them as a very useful diagnostic framework.

These ideas were once valued in our own culture — in the medieval world people were categorized into personality archetypes relating to the dominant element they manifested. Indeed, this concept was so mainstream that Shakespeare says in *Henry V*, 'He is pure air and fire; and the dull elements of earth and water never appear in him.'

The psychotherapist and psychologist Carl Jung also based many of his ideas relating to personality on the influence of elements upon the psyche — Air, for instance, related to thinking and intellect, Water to emotion and feelings, Earth to sensation, and Fire to intuition. The elements are also represented in the ancient principles of alchemy, which also have great correlation with the stages leading up to death.

The Earth element, which also relates to the bones and our inner vitality, is usually the first to go. The Water element then recedes and the skin, lips and eyes become parched and the emotions become unstable. When the Fire stage arrives with its burning fevers and chills, there may be vivid dreams of smoke and flying sparks, and very subtle changes to sight and vision. Finally, the Air element withdraws and there is difficulty breathing, the mind wanders and there is a gradual disconnection from the physical world.

EARTH

- *The Earth element is linked to our flesh and bones*

- *Chakra: Base*

- *Colour: Ochre*

- *Sense affected: Smell*

Physical Signs

The person will complain of great weariness and lack of joy for life. There may be aches and pains in the limbs and bones. They may feel nauseous and repelled by certain familiar smells, but may yearn for others. The carer may even notice a change of smell in the patient's, breath, skin or excretions. The complexion fades and takes on a greyish hue. The patient may be feeling very drained of energy. They may find it difficult to get out of bed, or to sit up. Strength to grasp objects diminishes and they may find it hard to keep a firm grip on objects such as cutlery. They often ask for extra pillows and for bedclothes to be removed because these feel too heavy against the skin.

Emotional Signs

They may become needy and tearful, and often don't like to be left alone for too long. May express a fear of silence and a fear of the dark.

Dreams and Sensations

These may vary between agitation and drowsiness, and the patient may mention dreams of shimmering mirages.

WATER

- *The Water element relates to blood, taste, liquids*

- *Chakra: Sacral*

- *Colour: Yellow*

- *Sense affected: Taste*

Physical Signs

The person may complain that food and drink tastes strangely different, perhaps sweeter or more acidic, dryer and rougher to the tongue. They may request specific foods such as boiled eggs, liver, paté on toast, and then feel nauseous when it arrives. There may be difficulty in moving the tongue, chewing and swallowing. Other signs include losing control of bodily liquids: nose runs, eyes water, dribbling from the corner of the mouth, incontinence, seepage from immobile limbs.

Emotional Signs

There may be a sensation of drowning, being pushed through water, heaviness, floating and sinking.

Dreams and Sensations

Their dreams may feature swirling wisps of smoke and an undulating haze, walking on water, swimming underwater.

FIRE

- *The Fire element relates to the major organs of the body: heart, lungs, liver and kidneys*

- *Chakra: Base*

- *Colour: Orange*

- *Sense affected: Sight (and 'vision')*

Physical Signs

There may be sudden and dramatic temperature fluctuations ranging from either shivering and trembling with cold to burning and wanting to kick off their bed coverings because of fever. During the cold phase the skin will look dry, sallow and parched. In the hot phase there may be vivid flushing. There may be excessive sweating, or sometimes no moisture in the skin at all. The lips become cracked and parched. The mouth and nose will dehydrate. The nose may bleed easily and profusely. Eventually as the phase gives way to the Air element, the feet and hands will start to feel cold as the warmth seeps away from the extremities and towards the heart. You may be able to feel a steamy heat rising from the crown chakra.

Emotional Signs

Shifts between clarity and confusion and eventually transformation to calm, detached acceptance.

Dreams and Sensations

Images of shimmering red sparks, sensation of panic and urgency. Restlessness, apprehension; they may feel a need to escape and get away from a 'brooding', menacing presence.

AIR

- *The Air element relates to the lungs and ears*

- *Chakra: Solar plexus*

- *Colour: Indigo*

- *Senses affected: Hearing and touch*

Physical Signs

Breathing becomes laboured and erratic. There may be rasping and panting and irregularity between breaths. Some breaths may appear to be missed altogether. The in-breaths may be short and snatched and the out-breaths weaker and longer. The death rattle may be present. Eyes may roll upwards or be tightly shut.

Emotional Signs

They may cry out, often in their sleep.

Dreams and Sensations

Hallucinations, visions, visits from dead relatives or enlightened beings, and talk of tunnels of light. Overwhelming sense of love and magnitude, insistent buzzing noises, flaming torches.

Other Important Signs That Death Is Approaching

There are other signs that also tell us when death is near. You will notice these perhaps two weeks or so before the end, when there is a shift from what doctors call the pre-active phase into the final active phase.

This final phase is marked by two distinct dynamics — the physical one, as the body begins to slowly shut down and die on a cellular level, and a spiritual one as consciousness and out-of-body-ness begins to expand.

No one can ever accurately predict how much longer someone has to live, even when they are in this final stage. The actual letting-go seems to be as much an emotional and spiritual decision as a physical release. Sometimes people rally for a while, in the final days acquiring a new strength and renewed enjoyment of life for a short time, while others move swiftly through it, withdrawing and growing steadily weaker. Drugs may also interfere with or mask some of these stages.

Decreasing Sociability

A slow withdrawal from wanting to take part in conversation and activity, which is partly due to increasing physical weakness. This often coincides with a reluctance to get out of bed. The patient may refuse visits from friends and relatives and seek the company of just one or two specific people.

Appetite Diminishes

This can cause real anguish for carers — who are demonstrating their love by cooking up tasty morsels — but refusing food at this stage is quite normal as the body becomes less able to digest food. Refusing food will not harm or hamper their progress. Offer and prepare what they would really like, such as a spoonful of mashed strawberries with cream, or a homemade fruit lolly — but don't be offended if it's left.

Agitation and Restlessness

These may manifest as agitation or the need to be moved or repositioned often. The patient may perform unusual repetitive actions such as plucking the bedcovers, complaining that pillows are uncomfortable or that the room is too hot/cold/noisy/draughty.

Increased Drowsiness and Changes in Speech and Consciousness

The patient may sleep for long periods, become muddled and appear to drift in and out of consciousness. They often mumble, reach out for invisible objects, laugh, twitch and make jerking movements.

Irregular Breathing

Rapid, shallow and intermittent breathing is normal in the final stages.

Poor Wound-healing

Wounds and infections may not heal as they used to and there may be persistent swelling, usually in the arms and legs.

Visions and Dreams and Language

Patients may describe seeing people who have already died, or speak about seeing or feeling the presence of loved ones or holy figures such as Jesus or the Buddha.

Sometimes your loved one might feel as if death is near and ask to talk about it and voice concerns about unfinished business.

Harold was one of the sweetest old men I had ever met. Kind, calm and always had little treats to give away to anyone who visited him. Twelve hours before he died he confided to one of the nurses who was bathing him that he had stood by and seen a child drown in a pond on the farm where he'd worked as a young man. He hadn't jumped in because he was scared of water. He'd kept it secret all his life but couldn't take it to the grave with him. He'd kept this terrible secret for nearly 70 years. So I just listened and we prayed together for the soul of the child and asked that God would forgive him.

Nina – hospice nurse

The Dying Room

One of the most poignant memories I have is of a man dying in a hospice as he suffered with the final stages of motor neurone disease. He was in his very final hours, and although beyond speaking was very acutely aware of what was happening, and also of his surroundings.

His family, who were on their way, had obviously made an effort to make the small private room as cosy as possible — the walls were covered with photographs and coloured drawings; they'd brought in their own blankets and cushions, and even plates, glasses and cutlery.

There was a large notice scribbled in blue felt pen on the wall next to a small CD player:

'Please put on a new CD from this collection for John — he so loves and needs to hear his favourite music — thank you.'

A beautiful antique cello was propped up next to his bedside table where a TV had been switched on and left blaring loudly. I quickly realized that the person who'd switched it on had left the room and obviously forgotten all about it.

This extremely sensitive man, who I later learned was a cellist of international repute, was dying to a background of noisy banter from Richard and Judy. It's a sad fact that many people are left to die with just a television on for company. Unless it's by choice, it must be very distressing being forced to endure the background noise of a loud radio or TV when you are too weak to protest.

In contrast, Suzi, who was having an almost near-perfect home death, always asked me the same question when I arrived to see her: 'How does the room feel?' She'd been in bed for weeks by then and wanted to know exactly how her visitors would feel walking into her room. It was a good question, as it forced me to tune in to the energies. It was always inviting, calm and clean and fresh-smelling.

Her illness was very advanced, yet she seemed to sparkle when friends arrived.

Her pretty bedroom, which was always filled with fresh flowers, felt very balanced and protective during her protracted illness, but in the last week it all changed — there was an air of almost palpable celebration about it as if a big party were being prepared. I wasn't sure how to convey this tactfully when Suzi asked again, just three days or so before she died, 'How does the room feel?' Although she was very weak by then she gave a huge smile when I replied enthusiastically, and said 'Good.' That's how it felt to her too, she said, and she felt almost giddy with joy and anticipation of whatever lay ahead of her.

FOR A GOOD ATMOSPHERE

- *Ensure that the room is clean, calm, clear and clutter-free.*

- *Bring the outside in: scented bulbs and blossom, scented garden flowers, orchids, shells, stones.*

- *Move the bed to ensure a good view of the outside if possible.*

- *Change sheets as often as possible — at least every other day.*

- *Add colour and comfort with lovely cushions, soft blankets, photographs, fabrics, cards.*

- *Provide a CD player or iPod (with headphones), a selection of music and talking books.*

- *Laptop, radio, torch.*

- *Aromatherapy oil-burner, candles. Selection of high-quality essential oils.*

- *Scented soaps, talcum powder, hand and body lotions.*

- *Provide large jigsaw puzzle (for visitors and children).*

Near-death Experiences

The idea that people can come back from the dead is completely commonplace in the East — it is a physical phenomenon called *Delogs*. These people reappear, having died and often been burned or buried for hours, days or weeks at a time, coming back as teachers to share their experiences within their community.

More and more people are being resuscitated and technically brought back from the dead after being in comas, or surviving heart attacks, and are telling very similar stories to the *Delogs*.

Near-death experiences (or NDEs as they are called) often include sensations of hearing strange buzzing noises and seeing tunnels of light. They may sometimes be attributed to disturbed brain chemistry (caused by drug treatment, for example), a lack of oxygen or changes in carbon dioxide levels. Of course, personal accounts do not constitute scientific proof, but the evidence does seem to show that consciousness and the mind may continue to exist after the brain has ceased to function and the body is clinically dead.

Dr Sam Parnia is one of the world's experts on NDEs. As well as being leader of the UK-based Consciousness Research Group, he is currently a fellow in Pulmonary and Critical Care Medicine at Weill Cornell Medical Centre, New York, and is Honorary Senior Clinical Research Fellow at the University of Southampton.

His groundbreaking work in studying NDEs is described in his book *What Happens When We Die*. Dr Parnia's team spent a year studying patients who had been successfully resuscitated following heart attacks and who, for a short time, had been clinically dead — with no pulse or respiration and with fixed, dilated pupils.

Only a relatively small number of patients in the trial had any vivid memories of emotions, sounds or visions during their period of unconsciousness, but as news of the study spread Dr Parnia received more than 500 testimonials from people who had survived close brushes with death.

Just like the patients in the study, they all described similar experiences:

- feelings of peace and joy

- heightened senses

- a sense of time being speeded up

- loss of body awareness

- seeing a bright light

- entering another world

- *reaching a definite point of no return.*

Interestingly, some people, a very small number, reported 'negative NDEs', often described as hellish, frightening and nightmarish, but unanimously the patients reported having experienced a 'spiritual journey', with an overall conviction that, once the final boundary was crossed, there would be no going back. Interestingly, nearly all of the people who described dying and returning said that their fear of death had been erased as a result of their experiences.

I found myself hovering above my body as the doctors struggled to get my heart going again, after a hysterectomy. I was astonished by the complete lack of emotion I felt — so this is what dying is about. No more emotional pain or anxiety any more. Freedom at last — I played around with this idea for a short while until I realized that it wasn't my time, and so I slipped back under my skin and back into my body again.

Jenny Hall

The Sacred Threshold

It used to be called arriving at 'death's door' — and it was the final threshold separating life from death.

Soul midwives honour it as a sacred threshold where heaven meets earth — a numinous zone which we all have to cross. As they work, they become temporary guardians of this space — holding it safely as the one they are guiding passes safely across.

The word 'sacred' means a place specially reserved for the worship and invocation of God or the gods. This threshold is certainly a place where a calling-in of the gods, for guidance and protection, may be our only way of navigating uncharted territory.

The mystics say it's where the 'veils are thin'; where we can, at certain times and in certain situations, stretch out and almost touch the invisible world beyond.

Many of us imagine it in archetypal images — a slow-flowing river, a chasm between crystal glaciers, a rainbow bridge, a place where the land, sea and sky meet. To me it's a whirling maelstrom where two mighty oceans merge.

This analogy of surging currents of water alludes to the sense of elemental power and challenge of the unknown that I feel when I am there escorting a dying friend. I am struck by its vastness, its strange sense of altered time, the unfamiliar boundaries that don't relate to any other recognizable physical or spiritual framework. It's magnificent — but not, in any way, compatible with life.

As death occurs, the spirit detaches from the body with a rapid sense of upward flight like a balloon taking off. But at the same time there is countering balance — a brooding, restless cloud of chaotic darkness. This is the doldrums of the deep soul, the bottom of its ocean bed as it anchors down, tethering itself to eternity.

The sacred threshold is both exquisitely light and claustrophobically dense, illuminated yet heavy — both ecstatic and sombre.

It is a very seductive place. With its extraordinary energies you can easily become very attached to its grand and ethereal unworldliness. Some soul workers have been there, and been tipped off-balance by its deep energies, and are reluctant to come home again; which is why only the most robust and grounded souls volunteer to accompany people there.

The Aura

Sombre, smooth, glowing, ragged or frazzled? Distinct or hazy? The first thing I notice when I walk into the room of someone who is dying is their aura.

Observing auras is a useful way of gauging how much time the dying person is spending 'out' of their bodies in preparation for leaving them finally. When someone is 'out' of their body their aura virtually disappears and it's as if they've just got a pilot light burning.

The aura, which is the outer protective energy sheaf around the physical body, is a very good measure of how someone is faring. It also tells me straight-away roughly how long we've got to work together, and how strong their life force, or *chi*, still is. It's like a barometer giving away so many vital clues.

The aura is made up of two parts — the Etheric, which is next to the skin, and the Energetic, which extends like a colourful plume around the body for about 40 cm. The two together tell us how strong the energy field is — and how it's being affected by the state of physical health, mental activity and emotional wellbeing.

The Etheric aura looks like a thin band of smoky grey film, with a misty outline about two cm wide. When we are awake it's compressed and thin, but during sleep or unconsciousness it expands to absorb universal *chi* energy and becomes noticeably softer and fuller.

When people are dying their auras change as each stage of death is completed. As the dying person grows weaker, the Etheric aura just starts fading away, very gradually, until it is almost undetectable — this also happens gradually with old age. But a couple of days before death, depending on the nature of the disease, the Etheric aura begins its rapid transformation, becoming softer and fuller. This is due to the chakras opening wide and discharging pulsating streams of heightened energy into the aura. This change can be seen, by sensitives, as a vivid luminous glow.

The Energetic aura is much wider than the Etheric and is seen around the body in swirling coloured bands. It has depth and texture, warm and cool areas, and parts of it tingle and dance with flashes of coloured light and streamers. These colours begin to fade and change slowly during the weeks before death. It diminishes until there is only a faint glow of colour left in it, giving it a pale hazy look. The Etheric aura (the thin smoky grey band next to the skin) also fades rapidly during this time.

The expansion of the Energetic aura, flooded by the energy from the chakras, often has the effect of temporarily revitalizing the dying person. It can also induce a heightened state of clairvoyance and clairaudience in varying degrees, enabling the dying to see across the sacred threshold and into the next world. They may also hear spirit voices and sounds.

Being surrounded by this energy can be very exhausting for carers, as it has a peculiar unnatural feel to it, a bit like a strong caffeine rush. You can become emotionally drained if exposed to it for even a short length of time, and it can manifest strange emotions ranging from extreme anxiety to anger and weepiness. Just for a time you are standing in the flow of energies that are emanating from a very powerful source, from this world and the other.

Dreams

The dreams of the dying often seem particularly muddled. But they are often loaded with symbolic imagery, giving useful glimpses into the inner labyrinth.

Dreams are the great tools for penetrating the psyche, linked as they are to unresolved issues, anxieties, forgotten themes and memories which may all need to be brought to closure, or at least acknowledged, before death.

Dreams, when understood as maps of our inner landscape, have a ingenious way of giving comforting knowledge to the dying. They bypass rational language and go straight to the heart of our understanding. They provide advance forays into the afterlife, and the subconscious mind seems to be always one step ahead in preparing the rational mind for death.

Stella, a farmer who was lingering in the pre-death stage, kept having the same dream. At her suggestion, we started a dream journal to unravel the messages within.

She dreamed she was locked in a house with a fire in it. She ran along the corridor locking all the doors to stop the fire spreading, but she could hear the roar of flames and feel the invading heat spreading up the walls — and then her feet became stuck. She couldn't move. When she thought with overwhelming panic that she was about to perish, a pigeon flew down the chimney and out from the fireplace, showing her that there was an escape route and fresh air beyond.

These images — and her particular choice of words as she recited the dream over and over again — really struck me with their vivid intensity: 'Stuck ... inferno ... breakthrough ... freedom'. I strongly sensed that these were nudges from Stella's own imagination showing her that she would be freed from the inferno and eventually escape to freedom and blue sky through a vertical shaft like a tunnel of light across to the world beyond.

As well as showing us our escape route, dreams can also be a way of introducing us to our guides or wise ones. It's very common for the dying to wake up and say they have been with Jesus, or an angel, or reunited with someone once close who has died, who appeared in order to act as an escort or psychopomp.

Dreams are often the portal into chaos and truth, and can be infused with huge significance for the dreamer. A strong dream can bring about huge shifts, swifter than hours of counselling might achieve. The intense messages and themes from dreams can bring great understanding, acceptance and relief from fear.

Pre-death dreams can also be cannily prophetic, as in the case of John Clarke, a butcher who woke up and perkily told his family that he had been talking to a lovely lady in a dream the night before, who'd told him he'd die 'a week on Thursday' — which proved to be absolutely right.

David, having worked as a Jungian psychotherapist for many years, requested that we use his on-going journal as a focus for our bi-weekly sessions. He illustrated his dreams in a sketchbook, using watercolour pencils, and it became clear that the dreams were an evolving narrative of images that symbolized the archetypal root of some of his strongest beliefs: 'I saw the hill where the great mother lived. It was strewn with fairy lights. A chink in the rock invited me in.' The following day David recalled that he'd been into the hill and found it to be full of animals and plants, and that he'd been tempted and invited to sample delicious foods.

Gradually he discussed a desire to go and live underground, inside the mother's breast (hill), knowing he would be safe and nurtured ... he also drew pictures of how his body actually 'felt' in his dreams, using different colours to illustrate his emotions and also to show where he was feeling soul pain as well as physical discomfort. By talking through these dream sequences, and looking back at them over a period of weeks, David was able to process many thoughts that were still just incubating, and eventually find peace of mind.

When I come to the end of the road
and the sun has set for me,
I want no tears in a gloom-filled room.
Why cry for a soul set free?
Miss me a little, but not too much,
and not with your head bowed low.
Remember the love that once we shared,
Miss me, but let me go.
This is a journey we all must take
and each must take alone;
It's all a part of God's perfect plan,
a step on the road to home.
When you are lonely and sick of heart,
go to the friends we know.
Bury your sorrows in doing good,
Miss me, but let me go.

Unknown

CHAPTER SIX
The Tool Kit

You'll find these items really useful as you sit and keep vigil at the bedside:

- *A soft shawl or very light blanket for swaddling or to give extra warmth and comfort if bedclothes are too heavy — preferably in beautiful, pastel colours (pinks, pale greens, blues). Mohair and cashmere are wonderful, although beware of anything too fluffy because loose fibres can fly all over the place, causing irritation.*

- *A cuddly toy. Many people, especially elderly people, like the reassurance of a very soft cuddly toy tucked up alongside them,* especially if they are missing their pets. They find it comforting to have something tucked in next to them if you have to leave the room for any length of time.

- Rescue Remedy. The spray version is very useful as it's safe and easy to administer and helps stressed carers as well as patients.

- Transition Essence. A simple energetic essence to help ease anxieties and help to ensure a peaceful death (see Flower Essences section, page 165).

- Crystals. Rose quartz to heal the heart and amethyst to bring harmony and dispel negativity.

- Essential oils either to burn in an oil-burner to fill the room with a therapeutic fragrance to aid sleep and refresh the air, or to mix with a carrier oil such as almond or avocado oil for massaging into hands or feet to bring relaxation and help with anxiety and pain relief. Specific oils:

- Sandalwood, which is traditionally used in Buddhist traditions to help the spirit leave the body after death.

- Rose oil to comfort the heart and balance the chakras.

- Chamomile to bring calm and help with breathing.

- Lavender to bring a sense of peace and encourage restful sleep.

- Tibetan singing bowls to create a soothing space. Their gentle but powerful tones work miracles and are healing for heart and mind. They will also purify a room after death and assist the dead person to go to the light.

- *Tingshaws (small Tibetan bells) to shift stagnant energy*

- *A bottle of holy water*

Crystals and Stones

Several years ago I stayed on the island of Eriska off the west coast of Scotland. It's so small that you can walk around its sandy beaches and circle the whole island in a morning.

The terrain is a mixture of bog and furze which stretches to the shore, merging seamlessly into sand, stone and seaweed. As I walked, my eyes scanned the tide mark for interesting shells, feathers and pebbles to take home, and there among the dark grey slate and sparkling schist stones I spotted a pink slab of rock, two hands wide, quite distinct from everything else.

It turned out to be a flat chunk of rough rose quartz — shaped, amazingly, like a human heart.

The smooth side had soft clefts, gouged out like the aorta and ventricles; on the other, rougher side there were coarse veins of green-blue quartz running from top to bottom. Astonishingly, there were no other similar stones on the island that I could see.

It felt as if I'd been meant to find it, and so I brought it home. It sits on a table in my sanctuary room absorbing the sunlight. It's an exquisite healing stone which radiates with the loving energy of the heart chakra. I now use it as a sort of battery charger for all my other healing stones, especially when they have been used to help people who are in a lot of pain.

These healing stones are various crystals and polished pebbles. They come in all shapes, sizes and colours. I use the amethyst and quartz geodes for energizing oils and essences and for absorbing negative energy, and the polished semi-precious stones for healing and therapeutic use.

They also work as talisman stones. If I have a patient who is very anxious or troubled by symptoms (such as insomnia) I set an 'intention' — a type of thought-form — around the stone to work with that person to help them with the problem that is distressing them. They keep the stone with them, under their pillow or beside their bed, and hold it when they need reassurance or healing. It's so simple, but so very comforting. I have several little polished hearts made of rose quartz which fit in the palm of the hand and my patients often hold them all night as they sleep. One or two patients have even asked to be buried with them.

Crystals are able to give out energy and receive it, and because of this it's essential to cleanse them properly before you use them (especially those that have been on display in shops, as they will have absorbed the energy of the shop). When you get them home, place them in salty water and leave them in the sun or moonlight for a couple of days.

Cleansing is also vitally important when using stones in between patients. I rest my crystals for weeks or even months by placing them out in the garden, in the sunshine, wind and rain to recharge them if they have helped people who are very sick.

If you choose to work with crystals you'll soon realize how independent and focused they are.

Sometimes a crystal only wants to work with one particular person who is dying and will request not to be put into use again. Honour its wish by taking it to the sea or a river and releasing it into the water.

The relationship with crystals is a completely co-operative one; there can be no sense of ownership with them. They know exactly how and when to do their work and will only stay with you for as long as they choose to. They sometimes mysteriously disappear and then reappear when you least expect them to. Sometimes they choose to go and live with someone else for a while and you simply have to let them go — with gratitude and appreciation for all the gifts they have brought you.

Here are the best gemstones for using with the dying. They can be used in the form of simple 'tumble-stones' or in their raw and unpolished state.

- *Clear quartz — one of the best all-round healing gemstones and psychic protectors.*

- *Smokey quartz — a grounding and general healing stone that works well combined with other gemstones. It helps people to 'let go' and can be programmed especially for transition work. Affinity: 5th and 6th chakras.*

- *Rose quartz — calming, and useful for opening the heart centre. It helps resolve emotional difficulties in allowing the clearing of difficult emotions and a fear of leaving people behind. Very good pain reliever. Affinity: 4th chakra.*

- *Amethyst — a very powerful healer! Also an excellent aid to meditation and spiritual matters. Helps to clear muddled minds. Has a balancing and calming effect. It also helps to lift the spirit and soothes aches and pains. Affinity: 6th chakra.*

- *Aquamarine — for grief, sadness and longing. Good for parents to use if sitting with a dying child. It has a very distinct angelic vibration and clarity. May aid inner understanding of difficult situations. Affinity: 7th chakra.*

- *Diamond — very good during radiotherapy and chemotherapy. If the immune system is severely depressed, place a diamond where* the cancer is manifesting. *Affinity: 7th chakra.*

- *Sodalite — works well on the throat and all related communication problems; encourages the wearer to 'speak and even acknowledge their truth' when they have had problems expressing difficult emotions. Affinity: 5th and 6th chakras.*

- *Amber — for breathing problems and panic attacks caused by breathlessness. Good also for 'getting things off your chest'. Affinity: 5th chakra.*

- *Adventurine — excellent in all matters physical or emotional and helps people adjust to uncertainty. Helps to open the heart chakra. Stimulates our connections with those around us. Affinity: 4th and 7th chakras.*

- *Hematite — for protection, especially from psychic attack! Very good for using in busy shared communal spaces (such as hospitals, especially high-dependency units where there may be a lot of shared anxiety within a small area). Good in cases of insomnia and for calming fevers, energizing and vitalizing. Also good for grounding and establishing a trusting relationship. Affinity: 1st chakra.*

- *Blue lace agate — a gentle balancing gemstone for body, mind and spirit. A help in cases of emotional exhaustion. A cooling gemstone to bring tranquillity. Affinity: 1st and 4th chakras.*

- *Amazonite — grounding and strengthening. Promotes clear thinking. Good for bringing a sense of closure. Stabilizes emotions. Affinity: 5th chakra.*

- *Snowflake obsidian — the healer's talisman. A powerful absorber of negative energy. Good for serious grounding and for protection. Needs very regular cleaning. Affinity: 1st chakra.*

- *Tiger's eye — promotes peaceful thoughts. Helps to calm anxiety and fear. Affinity: 2nd, 3rd and 5th chakras.*

- *Rhodonite — helps repair soul wounds and boost self-confidence. It's also said to improve the sharpness of the senses, especially hearing and listening. Affinity: 1st chakra.*

- *Jasper — helps to balance physical energies and strengthen the immune system. Promotes tissue regeneration and general healing. Affinity: 1st chakra.*

The knower of the mystery of sound knows the mystery of the whole universe.

Hazrat Inayat Khan

Music – a Massage for the Soul

There will come a time when a diseased condition will not be described as it is today by physicians and psychologists, but it will be spoken of in musical terms, as one would speak of a piano that was out of tune.

Rudolf Steiner

Aristotle and Plato both wrote about the healing power of music. During medieval times, a tradition of healing monastic chant for the sick developed. The Benedictine Order, which embraced holistic communal living, supported their sick or dying community members through the use of formal musical rituals. Sound is a physical phenomenon and directly affects our physiology. It is also able to affect the emotions by altering our brainwave from alpha to theta states (in a similar way to meditation), as well as potentially altering the vibration of our cells.

Music helps people to connect with their inner state and can help by alleviating pain, anxiety, nausea and insomnia. It can also help to release buried emotions and unlock memories, transforming their mood from anxious to calm.

The human voice is a powerful healing instrument and one that we all possess. Singing, humming, chanting are all techniques that we can bring to the bedside. According to the therapists who work with the voice in hospices, people can be tuned and brought back into harmony just like a musical instrument — by singing the right sequence of notes.

Of course, you need to be an expert to know exactly how to do this, but low humming or chanting can be very soothing if someone is in pain.

Jennifer spent two days at the bedside of her brother. 'I started singing all the lullabies and childhood songs that our mother sang to us to get us off to sleep — it worked like magic and made us both feel safe like babes again.'

Certain instruments can also be healing:

HARPS

Harps are often used in hospices. Music thanatology is a therapy based around the melodious sound and vibrational resonance of the harp — and is practised throughout many hospitals and hospices across the world. Although therapists use the harp for different effects, one of the main benefits is helping people to get their breathing back into a comfortable rhythm, especially after a panic attack or if they are having trouble with sleeping.

LYRES

The modern lyre, a small, harp-like instrument is becoming very popular as a healing aid, recalling the days when lyres were used in temples and traditionally associated with healing and spirituality. The ancient Greeks would prescribe one specific note to be played on the lyre to heal an illness. They are lovely to use and easy to handle as they're very portable and anyone can play them, just by randomly gliding their fingers over the strings.

SINGING BOWLS OR TIBETAN BELLS

These have been used by Tibetan monks for thousands of years for their meditative qualities and also for rebalancing the subtle bodies (see auras). I have been using singing bowls in my practice with great success and am constantly amazed at how they seem to make people adjust to difficult situations.

I work with two — one tuned to the note of F, which corresponds to the heart chakra, and one tuned to F sharp (and used to help people with the pain of a broken heart — which, for many of the older people I work with, has been endured and left unaddressed for almost a lifetime).

Besides their beauty, there is something quite other-worldly and ethereal about them. Their traditional uses are still bathed in secrecy and intrigue, having been known for their powerful effects in everything from summoning deities to clearing temples and homes of bad energy with their sonorous tones.

TINGSHAWS

These are small cymbals which you can bang together to shift stagnant energy. Ring them in the corners of the room to freshen up the atmosphere.

Therapists also use them by 'sounding' them over the chakra points to see where there are energy blockages. If they ring over a blockage the sound will change and become distorted.

As sound therapist Luane Crealy explains:

I always try to have a couple of sessions with my patients using the singing bowls. They help me get straight to the core of a person; we will share a deep silence for as long as the tone lasts. Sometimes the patient enters into an expanded state of consciousness, sometimes they fall asleep, and other times they may feel like talking, sharing memories or expressing previously contained emotions.

I felt as if an angel's wing had caressed my face, and suddenly I felt cleansed and whole again.

Sarah Frey

Flower Essences

From snowy Alaska to the arid Australian Bush, flower remedies have been a traditional part of almost every culture's pharmacopoeia.

Most of us are familiar with the Bach Flower Remedies, which were created by Harley Street physician and homoeopath Dr Edward Bach in the 1930s.

Roaming the English country lanes he intuitively collected 38 specimens of native plants and trees and made a collection of energetic essences from them by soaking them in spring water outside in the sunlight, following a homoeopathic method. His famous Rescue Remedy, which is a blend of five plants, is still a bestseller.

Dr Bach was convinced that negative emotions were the root of physically manifesting disease and that long-term feelings such as shyness, jealousy and fear could eventually make us ill, if left unresolved. Each of his remedies is designed to shift these states of mind.

Some people react to flower remedies astonishingly quickly and are able to release layers of emotional debris in just a couple of days.

Alicia had been a traditional herbalist for most of her working life and was also very skilled in making flower remedies. After discovering that she had terminal cancer of the kidney, she spent several weeks during her last summer making remedies for her many friends and relatives from the infused petals of forget-me-nots. Tiny blue bottles of the exquisite essence made by her were handed out at her funeral as therapeutic keepsakes.

MAKING FLOWER REMEDIES

Flower remedies, like gem essences, are easy to make and easy to use.

Flower lore says that the plants that are growing in our own back gardens are usually the ones that have come to heal us. It's worth seeing what's out there and what hints they are dropping.

Soak freshly gathered flower heads in fresh spring water, in a glass or crystal bowl, out in the sun for several hours. Strain them and pour the infusion into clean pipette-topped bottles with a drop of brandy or cider vinegar to preserve.

Be certain to use flowers that you know to be safe. As a rule only use blossoms that you know to be edible such as roses, marigolds, nasturtiums, violets and edible herbs.

The essences are either taken directly onto the tongue, or in water. If the person you are treating isn't able to swallow, place a few drops into the tummy button or spray around them using a clean atomizer.

Some useful commercial remedies:

- *Cherry plum — obsessive fear, nervous exhaustion and fear about losing control*

- *Agrimony — for those who are cheerful and confident on the outside but hide anxiety and mental torture within*

- *Rose — wonderful for soothing broken hearts. It's also very helpful for relatives coming to terms with loss*

- *Honeysuckle — for those clinging to the past and who are in denial about their illness*

- *Heather — loneliness, withdrawal and melancholy. Can be useful with confused and elderly patients*

- *Rescue Remedy — a marvellous cure-all in times of stress.*

My favourite homemade essences include:

- *Angelica — helps to promote calm after shock or turmoil. Helps create a connection to the patient's spirit guides and helpers*

- *Nasturtium — for spiritual attunement and nervous exhaustion*

- *Marigold — for harnessing the energy of the sun and for healing burn-out*

- *Jasmine — linking to higher bodies and strengthening the aura*

- *Rosemary — enhancing memory*

- *Thyme — for adjusting to inner and outer body experiences*

- *Borage — for courage.*

Essential Oils

Nothing stimulates the senses quicker than the power and joy of smell. Essential oils made from aromatic plants work on body and mind, encouraging healing at a subtle level, as well as encouraging a positive outlook. Used regularly, the oils promote calm and tranquillity, and most people really enjoy them.

The oils created from flowers, bark, leaves and fruit are so highly concentrated and aromatic that they are said to represent the inner soul of the plant and its synergistic relationship to the sun — no wonder they have such an affinity with the human psyche. They bombard the senses with pure unadulterated healing power.

Many essential oils also have intense antiseptic properties, far stronger than some of their commercial equivalents. For example, the oils of lemon, thyme, oregano and cloves are all capable of killing typhoid and diphtheria when administered in the appropriate dose. These properties make them extremely useful in the sick room, where they can be used in burners or diluted with water in spray to clear and sweeten the air.

- Petitgrain — tranquillizer, good for anxiety and depression.

- Rose — soul wounds, good for women, good for broken hearts, grief, jealousy, anxiety.

- Lavender — many spiritual and therapeutic qualities which soothe the emotions.

- Chamomile — calming, helps relaxation and meditation, nervousness and difficult behaviour.

- Rosewood — protects centredness, eases the mind, helps connect with loved ones and carers, good for stress. Can stabilize energy levels. Good for restless minds.

- *Frankincense — sets the spirit free. Spiritual and religious, holding negative energies at bay. Expands consciousness. Sacred associations. Heals old wounds. Good for paranoia and nightmares. Helps inward reflection.*

- *Sandalwood — courage, stabilizes mind/ body/spirit, alleviates loneliness and obsessiveness.*

- *Lemon myrtle — energy shifts, antiseptic, emotional uplift.*

- *Geranium — warm, nurturing, loving, balances highs and lows; in uncertainty it will guard against excessive sensitivity.*

- *Myrrh — deep connection to spirit, endurance and strengthening. Promotes inner silence, allows for processing of difficulties.*

Gem Essences

Gem essences have been revered as powerful remedies in Ayurvedic medicine for more than 10,000 years. Some of the prescriptions described in the Vedas for tinctures and salves and oral medicines involving crushed lapis lazuli and rubies are still in use by some practitioners today.

Modern experts say that gem therapy sits somewhere between homeopathy and the flower remedies because it works by linking emotions with the physical body, using the vibrational field of the gemstones to harmonize with the dis-eased field of the patient.

Modern computer technology relies on the potency of minute quartz crystals to transmit electrical transmissions, and there is research in Russia examining the force fields of the crystals and their ability to affect the electromagnetic field within the atoms and molecules in our bodies.

Photographs using Kirlian cameras which show the human aura — the body's energy field — show how specific crystals are able to strengthen the aura when placed close to or on the body. Simply speaking, gems work like tuning forks on parts of the body that are diseased or out of balance

Crystals and gems can also absorb radiation and protect us from harmful rays — it's useful to have a few amethysts in your pocket if you are having to spend hours in a hospital where there is electromagnetic radiation from equipment, computers and phones, etc.

Gem remedies are easy to make and are another useful ingredient in the tool kit.

MAKING GEM REMEDIES

1. *First, clean the gem under running water and leave it in the sun for several hours if you can, to soak up healing energy.*

2. *Then place the gem in a one-pint glass or crystal dish filled with fresh spring water and leave to soak for up to 24 hours.*

3. *Remove it with a clean spoon and decant into a labelled dark bottle with a teat stopper.*

To Use

Mix four drops of gem essence to a tablespoon of water and take whenever required.

GEM OILS

Follow the same method as above but soak the gems in oil rather than water.

Use the oil for anointing or massage and mix with essential oils for a scented version.

Gem Aura Spray

This can be very useful for cleansing or revitalizing a room or for spraying close to someone who isn't able to swallow.

Fill an atomizer spray with your chosen gem remedy, adding essential oils or flower remedies if required.

You can spray these direct around the aura, pulse points, spaces or direct onto the body.

Holy Water

Our native rivers and springs are the arteries of the earth; and the waters that flow through them have been celebrated for centuries for their healing powers.

Using water for use in healing is an idea that is still an active tradition within the Church, and it's one that I like. Holy water isn't technically 'holy' unless it's been consecrated by a priest or bishop, but anyone can bless and honour water and celebrate its life-giving properties of conferring blessings, invoking healing energy and dispersing negativity.

One man, a professional homoeopath, dedicates his life to dispersing holy water over the motorways of England, especially along accident black spots. It's his act of service to the planet. He makes a huge barrel every weekend and drives hundreds of miles, sprinkling it along the fast lane from the back of his van.

1. *To make your own holy water, fill a clean bowl with fresh spring water. Centre yourself with a prayer and using your right hand raised above the bowl, invite divine universal energy to flow through you and into the water.*

2. With your left hand, make the sign of a circle with a cross inside it (or a symbol belonging to the tradition you're aligned to). Hold the image in your mind for several moments and ask for the water to be filled with healing and love. The water will then be charged and filled with dynamic energy.

Here is the traditional Catholic prayer for blessing water, which can be said over the bowl:

God, who for the salvation of the human race has built Your greatest mysteries upon this substance, in Your kindness hear our prayers and pour down the power of Your blessing into this element, prepared by many purifications. May this Your creation be a vessel of divine grace to dispel demons and sicknesses, so that everything that it is sprinkled on in the homes and buildings of the faithful will be rid of all unclean and harmful things. Let no pestilent spirit, no corrupting atmosphere, remain in those places: may all the schemes of the hidden enemy be dispelled. Let whatever might trouble the safety and peace of those who live here be put to flight by this water, so that health, gotten by calling Your holy name, may be made secure against all attacks. Through the Lord, amen.

Many people possess a bottle of holy water from Lourdes, the river Jordan or a revered holy well as spiritual talisman. You can use the water to bathe and bless them. I revere the sparkling and icy cold water from the Chalice Well at Glastonbury, which is very soft and feminine and known for its miraculous restorative powers involving sight and expanding spiritual vision.

As you tune in to different waters you will sense the different energies between them, and will begin to intuitively know when to use them. You may have a holy well waiting to be revived and used in your own town or village.

Use the water freely. It holds its potency for a few days, and when you finish with it return it back into the earth, with thanks. Or do as I do: water your plants with it.

First there must be order and harmony within your own mind. Then this order will spread to your family, then to the community and finally to your entire kingdom. Only then can you have peace and harmony.

Confucius

Stilling the Mind

Bring your mind home. And release. And relax.

Tibetan Book of Living and Dying

Worry, exhaustion and fear may hamper the journey for both patient and carer.

Knowing how to centre ourselves and access an inner sanctuary of calm strengthens us when the going gets tough.

Meditation gently applies the brakes to our mind, to silence the inner chatter when our thoughts are running out of control.

The beauty of meditation is that it's relatively simple to learn; anyone, young or old, can do it. You don't have to be religious or spiritual to learn how to use it.

Many doctors recommend simple mediation exercises to help treat chronic pain, and many clinical studies have shown that it can reduce levels of pain as well as easing panic attacks, lowering blood pressure and breathing and pulse rates.

One of the ways that it works is by restoring the balance between the emotional and thinking parts of the brain. We can do this by concentrating on our breath or by focusing on an object such as a candle flame, or by using a repetitive sentence — like a mantra — which stills the mind.

THE KEY TO MEDIATION IS RELAXATION

Plan to set aside half an hour with no interruptions. Switch off the phone and find a warm, safe and quiet place to be. Wrap yourself in a warm blanket for extra comfort. When you are settled and comfortable, gently close your eyes.

Spend a few moments tuning in to how you are feeling both physically and emotionally. Then beginning with your toes, concentrate on the different areas of your body up to your head, sensing how your body is feeling. You may find tension, tightness, tingling, heat, etc.

Gradually bring your attention back to your breathing and 'watch' as the breath enters and leaves your body. Be aware of the movement of your breath, the flow and the rhythm as it gently enters and leaves your body. Don't try to change the rhythm, just be aware of it and any feelings that arise.

Now let the breath flow and simply breathe. If thoughts flood into your mind, just let them come and go again but keep returning to the pattern of your breathing, letting it flow in and out with each moment.

Notice the pause and stillness between each breath — in and out. Now, silently count at the moment of stillness just before each in-breath up to a count of five ... breathe out — count one, breathe in, breathe out — count two, breathe in, breathe out — count three, breathe in, breathe out — count four, breathe in, breathe out — count five, breathe in ... continue repeating this. If you become distracted, gently bring your focus back to the count and begin again from one.

Acknowledge any thoughts or feelings that arise, but don't analyse them. Simply let them go.

Some people prefer to repeat a mantra or phrase to calm the mind instead of counting, or imagine themselves walking through a beautiful garden or stepping into a waterfall to calm the mind.

As you bring the meditation to an end, bring your focus back to your breathing and gradually become aware of your body again. Then, when you are ready, gently open your eyes and take a few minutes to reflect on the experience.

CHAPTER SEVEN
When Death Comes

*When all goes well there is a crystalline quality that emerges
which everyone in the room can feel, like a symphony that lifts
the soul.*

*What arises from these depths and cannot be measured is
guided by an invisible hand that finds its mark.*

*What could not be accomplished separately becomes available
to those who work together and the wholeness that surfaces in
these moments is characterized by luminous transparency.*

Christopher Bache, Dark Night Early Dawn

Energy Shifts

The energy in the room changes as death approaches
and you will know that it is time to create a tranquil
atmosphere in preparation for the last phase.

It's important now to remove all sources of sensory stimulation including scented flowers, incense, and music (which may lead to attachment). Switch off the electric lights (or replace lightbulbs with soft orange or pink coloured ones instead) and light plain white candles instead).

As you sit or lie beside your friend, be aware of the subtle energy changes as they happen.

This final stage so often seems to happen at night as the body's natural rhythms slow down and prepare for sleep, and this can be a long session of waiting, watching and knowing. Being there to lovingly assist and hold the space for whatever needs to unfold, is our sacred role.

Practise deep listening, contemplation and mindfulness within yourself and check that you are centred and feeling grounded and secure. You may intuitively find yourself entering the Dream State of your friend and will be able to guide them on their way. If you haven't prepared this with them in advance, just whisper in their ear to follow the light and let them know that they will be greeted by someone who will come especially to meet them.

You may start to be notice the four elements withdrawing from the body, if they haven't done so already. If you have been vigiling you will probably have sensed, over the last few days, that your friend has been spending moments, sometimes even prolonged periods, outside their body as their link with life and the physical grows weaker.

There may be a death-rattle sound as liquid gathers in the throat and chest, which can sound unpleasant but it isn't usually distressing for the person dying. Soothe and calm them by speaking gently, or singing their name and assuring them as much as you can that everything is well and that there is nothing at all to fear.

At this stage repetitive phrases or poems are comforting. I love and often use the words of Julian of Norwich, the 14th-century mystic who comforted all those she encountered in anguish by saying: 'All shall be well, and all shall be well and all manner of things shall be well.' I often whisper it over and over again as a comforting mantra.

Be mindful for your friend and everything that they are experiencing both physically and beyond the realms of human understanding. They may especially be feeling panic, and struggling to get enough oxygen, they may have a strong fear of the enveloping darkness, and a resistance to let go and surrender. But gradually you'll sense that a feeling of peace is descending and that slowly and gently they are beginning to loosen their grasp on life and are becoming ready to let go.

As you sit with them you can help by:

- *gently encouraging them to let go of their breath — sometimes it can help to say that you will breathe for them*

- *telling them how much they are loved, how much they have been loved and how safe they are*

- *encouraging them to gently go, giving permission if you feel that you need to and if it feels helpful*

- *assuring them that they will not be alone, or frightened, that they will be loved and greeted as they make the transition.*

There are powerful forces at work at this time. Be aware that just before the intake of the last breath, but not necessarily at the point of death, the soul goes into a place of unconditional love, and has the opportunity to deal with all unfinished business while often experiencing a series of life reviews.

The dying person will begin their rapid expansion into awareness. And as they take their last breath (which you may not notice if their breathing has been very irregular) you will sense that their body is emptying and becoming hollow as the life force ebbs away.

Sometimes, just in the final moments before death, even if the person has been semi-conscious and sleepy for hours on end, they will suddenly open their eyes wide, move or try to sit up and may look as if they have seen a vision. Don't be alarmed if this happens — one old man who'd been a rag-and-bone man all his life woke up startled but overjoyed just moments before his death and shouted 'Walter' — his daughter recognized it as being the trusty and dearly loved horse that had, for many years, pulled his cart.

The shift of energy when death finally happens can feel rather like an explosive firework going off and there can be noticeable shock waves in the room.

This is often followed by a vacuum force that sucks the vitality from the room, including all the warmth within it. A sudden chill may descend and the air and space around the dead person can feel very cold. The atmosphere in the room (depending on the nature of the death) may feel very disturbed for several days.

When you have come to the edge of all the light you know,
and are about to step off into the darkness of the unknown,
faith is knowing that one of these two things will happen:
there will either be something solid to stand on
or you will be taught how to fly.

Anonymous

Looking After Ourselves

Looking after people who are dying is intensely emotionally and physically exhausting, however much we love them.

On an energetic level, very seriously ill people often seem to absorb the vitality of those around them, as if to boost their own diminishing supplies, and many professionals and healers who specialize in working with the very seriously ill often have very short working lives — in terms of the amount of work they can do year-in and year-out.

Most of us feel very depleted and hollow after being at the bedside of someone who is dying — sometimes it's the effects of grief, but it can also be a sign that we should return to ourselves and honour our own need to heal and be kind and loving to ourselves.

Listen when your own wise self tries to tell you to take time out to nurture and revitalize — sometimes we just don't heed the warnings.

I loved the idea of a colleague of mine when he said,

I really need to have some sort of petrol gauge on the palm of my hand to let me know when I'm in danger of running on an empty tank — when I'm about to go down below my own safe reserves. If I don't stop in time and see the signs, I can feel totally drained and exhausted for weeks.

Within any carer/patient/healer relationship there's a need to recognize your own limits in terms of how much energy you give out. When you sit with an open heart it's all too easy to forget to seal yourself up and refresh yourself after a long session.

Soul midwives recognize this and will consciously prevent this happening by strengthening their own energy field before working and cleansing themselves after a session.

There are many rituals that healers follow, such as imagining themselves bathing under cascading fountains, or bathing in a blue light just as doctors always used to wash their hands in between patients.

This practice was partly to prevent disease spreading but also a symbolic cleansing of their own energy field.

A room filled with the energy of a sick person may get very toxic, sticky and stagnant, and the energy may really benefit everybody by regular cleansing on an energetic level.

There are many traditional ways of doing this, from burning sage bundles to sprinkling salt into the four corners of the room, to toning with voice or singing bowls, clapping hands, using Tingshaws and spraying with essential oils or essences.

If you are spending a lot of time with someone who is dying, make extra sure that you look after your own needs as much as possible.

Eat well, as much fresh food as possible, get as much sleep as you can. Take time out to see friends, take as much fresh air and sunlight as possible, do yoga or Tai Chi, dancing, singing, etc.

All these activities, besides boosting your energy levels, will help to bring you back into balance again and stop you from burning out.

Recognize when you are tired or under par and withdraw for a little while. You have to be in very good shape to help others.

Remember: we are the most important people in our own lives and we need to learn how to take care of ourselves.

If you are looking after someone who is ill or dying, you will be able to do more for them if you love and care for yourself:

- do some gardening

- take a walk in the countryside

- have a swim

- go for a massage

- *take a scented bath in candlelight*

- *bake bread or a cake*

- *paint a picture*

- *put some music on and dance*

- *sing.*

Reclaiming Our Energy

Chanting, or singing your own name, is an ancient shamanic method in reclaiming your energy when others have either consciously or unconsciously connected to you.

Begin by saying your name aloud, saying, 'I am and only [say your name]. There is no one within or connected to me that is not [say your name again]'. Say it with clear intent, and feel it resonate deep inside.

This technique is very good if you feel spacey and exhausted and will help you feel strong and clear again.

After Death

When someone has been in my care, I always carry on talking to them after they have died. It may just be for four or five hours, sometimes it's much longer, perhaps a week or so but usually it's for about three days until I feel that they are no longer there.

Many traditions recognize the period between death and burial as sacred and there are many rituals, both private and collective, which can be held to honour this time.

One of the most beautiful practices is anointing and washing the body to prepare for burial — it can be one of the most devotional acts of love to perform. The symbolic meaning of anointing is to prepare and nourish the body and soul for the onward journey and it was usually performed by family members, especially the women, who would share the task.

Preparing your own anointing oil is an act of grace in itself — I make mine using a base of sweet almond oil which has been infused with angelica, rosemary, rose, sandalwood and myrrh.

If I am not able to be with the person who has died, perhaps because they have died far away, I will light a candle and pray that they are safe and have been met by someone who loves them. You can do this simple ritual for someone even years after the death has occurred. Occasionally I have worked with women who have miscarried babies and never properly grieved for them — sometimes 50 years after the event.

IN THE DAYS FOLLOWING DEATH

Slowly and peacefully return the loving focus back to yourself. Be especially gentle and take your time to sit quietly. Don't be rushed into saying goodbye too quickly, which is something that you may regret later. Just sit in the silence, reflecting on all you have experienced.

The days following death will bring their own gifts — see this as a pause from normal life, a time for deep reflection, a time for forgiveness, a time to plan anew and an opportunity to take a long view of life before we become busy and distracted again.

Even the longest night eventually ends with dawn and the piercing of the first golden dawn light reminds us that a new day has begun. Yesterday is a memory, tomorrow still a dream; today we are here in the present with our own precious lives to live.

Do not stand at my grave and weep,
I am not there; I do not sleep.
I am a thousand winds that blow,
I am the diamond glints on snow,
I am the sunlight on ripened grain,
I am the gentle autumn rain.
When you awaken in the morning's hush,
I am the swift uplifting rush
Of quiet birds in circling flight.
I am the soft starlight at night.
Do not stand at my grave and cry,
I am not there; I did not die.

attributed to Mary E Frye

AFTERWORD

In the time that it has taken you to read this book, thousands of people across the planet will have taken their last breath and died. And many of those left behind will be grieving and perhaps wishing they had been able to do more for their loved ones. But, as we have seen, there are so many different ways that we can help the dying and their passing.

Plato had the idea that every soul who comes to earth has been 'called' here. Living is certainly about experiencing who and what we are, and both experimenting and enjoying this great adventure that we call life. I feel it's also about inspiring and encouraging others to be themselves and helping them to live their lives to the full. Dying is nothing more than an ending of this earthly sojourn, and I believe, as many do, that when it's over we're 'called' home again.

Imagine if the thin veils that separate the invisible world and its vibrant community of ancestors from ours were to disappear. What would it be like if we could catch sight of what lies ahead of us? Would it dissolve our fear of death for ever?

I think it would. As we all step closer towards the light, the extraordinary truth of who we are and our part in the divine plan would become clear, and death would finally be seen for the great illusion it is.

In helping people to make the transition between this life and the next, I feel so heartened by what I have seen and heard. Time after time I've been certain that there are love and joy waiting for everyone as they arrive home again. For me, this tiny view of the life beyond is the greatest reward for being someone's soul companion while they die.

So if you are helping someone you love on their way, remember that their soul is always their truest and greatest guide. As companions, we are simply there to hold the map, slip a comforting arm around them and shine the torch to enable them to clearly see the pathway ahead.

With all blessings and love,

Felicity Warner

June 2008

APPENDIX

If someone is dying at home, all the ideas in this book are simple and easy enough to perform and you have autonomy in all that you do.

If the death takes place away from home, however, and you are hoping to vigil, anoint or prepare the body after death, you will need to co-operate with the hospital, hospice or care home where the death takes place. It is advisable to mention any unusual wishes to the care team well in advance so that preparations can be made as soon as possible.

While the person is alive, they have the authority to have their wishes respected and accommodated. In order for the wishes to be binding, though, the person may have to write them down in an advance directive document, such as a statement of wishes or a living will. This can be done in the presence of a solicitor or GP to make it extra watertight.

Once the person has died, the rights regarding their body transfer to their closest relatives. No one 'owns' a body as such, but hospitals, etc. will have their own rules and regulations as to what should happen to a body while it's under their care.

Official institutions vary considerably in their approaches; some will be more accommodating than others. In my experience, tact and courtesy really help here.

If you are hoping to use essential oils, sound therapy, therapeutic touch, singing or chanting whilst you care for your loved one, you will need to co-operate fully with the nursing staff and explain to them what you are doing and what it will entail.

Most hospitals have a flexible multi-faith care policy that facilitates religious or important cultural rituals (such as enabling Romany people to die in an outside area if requested). For guidance, talk to the ward team, the team social worker and also the hospital chaplain.

Many wards in hospitals have a single room attached which may be suitable for vigiling, so it's worth asking if this is available.

Hospices or care homes usually have greater flexibility to accommodate personal preferences.

But fulfilling someone's wishes will still probably involve prior discussion and planning with the staff, co-operation and some flexibility on your part.

If you wish to wash and anoint the body of your loved one, you will need to do this up to about four hours or so after the death and before rigor mortis sets in. Tell the staff well ahead of time that this is important to the person and is something you plan to do. Many hospitals will help you achieve this if you give them enough notice — sometimes a room may be provided or, alternatively, the hospital chapel may be made available for a short time.

If this isn't possible, there may still be an opportunity to anoint the body when it has been removed and taken to the undertakers (they will be able to prepare it in order for you to comfortably perform this final act with your loved one), either on their premises or by helping you to bring the body home again.

If you wish to bring the body home for the period between death and the funeral, you will need to organize refrigeration equipment and professional help in handling, preparing and storing the body. Many undertakers will assist you with this, but you need to enquire ahead of time and contact a number of possible undertakers to ensure that you find one that can definitely help you with your plans.

For advice on these matters, contact the Natural Death Centre in London. The staff there are marvellous at helping with all these issues. Their helpline is manned for immediate enquiries for several hours a day — telephone 0871 288 2098 or write to The Natural Death Centre, 12a Blackstock Mews, Blackstock Road, London N4 2BT or email via their website www.naturaldeath.org.uk.

Hay House Titles of Related Interest

YOU CAN HEAL YOUR LIFE, the movie,
starring Louise L. Hay & Friends
(available as a 1-DVD set and an expanded 2-DVD set)

Watch the trailer at www.LouiseHayMovie.com

****

You Can Heal Your Life, by Louise L. Hay

The Healing Power of Nature Foods,
by Susan Smith Jones PhD

Through My Eyes, by Gordon Smith

What Happens When We Die, by Dr Sam Parnia

We hope you enjoyed this Hay House book.
If you would like to receive a free catalogue featuring additional
Hay House books and products, or if you would like information
about the Hay Foundation, please contact:

Hay House UK Ltd
292B Kensal Rd • London W10 5BE
Tel: (44) 20 8962 1230; Fax: (44) 20 8962 1239
www.hayhouse.co.uk

***

Published and distributed in the United States of America by:
Hay House, Inc. • PO Box 5100 • Carlsbad, CA 92018-5100
Tel.: (1) 760 431 7695 or (1) 800 654 5126;
Fax: (1) 760 431 6948 or (1) 800 650 5115
www.hayhouse.com

Published and distributed in Australia by:
Hay House Australia Ltd • 18/36 Ralph St • Alexandria NSW 2015
Tel.: (61) 2 9669 4299; Fax: (61) 2 9669 4144
www.hayhouse.com.au

Published and distributed in the Republic of South Africa by:
Hay House SA (Pty) Ltd • PO Box 990 • Witkoppen 2068
Tel./Fax: (27) 11 467 8904 • www.hayhouse.co.za

Published and distributed in India by:
Hay House Publishers India • Muskaan Complex • Plot No.3
B-2 • Vasant Kunj • New Delhi – 110 070.
Tel.: (91) 11 41761620; Fax: (91) 11 41761630.
www.hayhouse.co.in

Distributed in Canada by:
Raincoast • 9050 Shaughnessy St • Vancouver, BC V6P 6E5
Tel.: (1) 604 323 7100; Fax: (1) 604 323 2600

***

Sign up via the Hay House UK website to receive the Hay House
online newsletter and stay informed about what's going on with
your favourite authors. You'll receive bimonthly announcements
about discounts and offers, special events, product highlights,
free excerpts, giveaways, and more!
www.hayhouse.co.uk

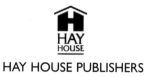